Animal Abuse and Family Violence: Linkages, Research, and Implications for Professional Practice

Animal Abuse and Family Violence: Linkages, Research, and Implications for Professional Practice has been co-published simultaneously as *Journal of Emotional Abuse*, Volume 7, Number 3 2007.

Animal Abuse
and Family Violence:
Linkages, Research,
and Implications
for Professional Practice

Marti T. Loring, PhD, LCSW
Robert Geffner, PhD, ABPN, ABPP
Janessa Marsh, MA
Editors

Animal Abuse and Family Violence: Linkages, Research, and Implications for Professional Practice has been co-published simultaneously as *Journal of Emotional Abuse,* Volume 7, Number 3 2007.

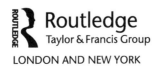

Routledge
Taylor & Francis Group

LONDON AND NEW YORK

First published 2007 by Haworth Press, Inc

Published 2018 by Routledge
52 Vanderbilt Avenue, New York, NY 10017
2 Park Square Milton Park, Abingdon Oxon OX14 4RN

Routledge is an imprint of the Taylor & Francis Group, an informa business

© 2018 by Taylor & Francis.

Notice:
Product or corporate names may be trademarks or registered trademarks, and are used only for identification and explanation without intent to infringe.

Cover design by Jennifer M. Gaska.

Library of Congress Cataloging-in-Publication

Animal abuse and family violence : linkages, research, and implications for professional practice /Marti T. Loring, Robert Geffner, and Janessa Marsh, guest editors.
p. cm.
"Co-published simultaneously as Journal of emotional abuse, volume 7, number 3 2007."
Includes bibliographical references and index.
ISBN-13: 978-0-7890-3818-0 (hard cover : alk. paper)
ISBN-13: 978-0-7890-3819-7 (soft cover : alk. paper)
1. Animal welfare. 2. Pets. 3. Family violence. I. Loring, Marti T. II. Geffner, Robert.

III. Marsh, Janessa. IV. Journal of emotional abuse.
HV4708.A5423 2007
179′.3–dc22

2007035067

ISBN13 - 9780789038180 (hbk)
ISBN13 - 9780789038197 (pbk)

ABOUT THE EDITORS

Marti T. Loring, PhD, LCSW, is a social worker and sociologist in Atlanta, Georgia. She is director of the Center for Mental Health and Human Development; and the Emotional Abuse Institute. Dr. Loring's expertise is in the areas of abuse and trauma. She has taught in several universities and conducted training seminars. She has written several articles published in professional journals and two books, including *Emotional Abuse*. An evaluator in court cases, Dr. Loring has testified across the country in cases including issues of animal abuse. Some of her research has involved the role of pet abuse in family violence; in particular, animal abuse as a means of coercion when battered women are forced into illegal acts.

Robert Geffner, PhD, ABPP, ABPN, is Founder and President of the Family Violence and Sexual Assault Institute in San Diego, CA; President of Alliant International University's Institute on Violence, Abuse and Trauma; Acting Director of Alliant's Center of Forensic Studies; Clinical Research Professor of Psychology at the California School of Professional Psychology, Alliant International University; Licensed Psychologist and Licensed Marriage & Family Therapist in California and Texas; Editor-in-Chief of Haworth's Maltreatment & Trauma Press, which also includes being the Editor of three internationally disseminated journals (*Journal of Child Sexual Abuse and Journal of Aggression, Maltreatment & Trauma*, and co-editor of *Journal of Emotional Abuse*); and former clinical director of a large private practice mental health clinic in East Texas for over 15 years. He has a Diplomate in Clinical Neuropsychology and one in Family Psychology. He served as an adjunct faculty member for the National Judicial College for 10 years, and was a former Professor of Psychology at the University of Texas at Tyler for 16 years. He has also been a researcher and consultant during the past 25 years. Publications include recent treatment manuals, edited books concerning family violence and child maltreatment, one book in press, and numerous book chapters, journal articles and research papers concerning family violence, sexual assault, child abuse, family and child psychology, custody issues, forensic psychology, neuropsychology and diagnostic assessment. He has also served on several national and state committees dealing with various aspects of family psychology, family violence, child abuse, and family law. He has presented over 450 keynote addresses, plenaries, workshops, and seminars at international, national, regional, and state conferences or meetings.

Janessa Marsh, MA, is Assistant Editor for the *Journal of Aggression, Maltreatment & Trauma*, the *Journal of Child Sexual Abuse*, the *Journal of Emotional Abuse*, and the new *Journal of Child and Adolescent Trauma* and is on staff at the Institute on Violence, Abuse and Trauma at Alliant International University in San Diego, CA. Ms. Marsh received her Master's Degree in Industrial-Organizational Psychology from the California School of Organizational Studies at Alliant International University and her undergraduate degree from Louisiana State University.

Animal Abuse and Family Violence: Linkages, Research, and Implications for Professional Practice

CONTENTS

POLICY AND PRACTICE

About the Contributors

Alonzo M. Cavazos, Jr., EdD, LCSW, is Associate Professor of Social Work at the University of Texas-Pan American. His research focuses on traditional healing among Latinos and on field instruction in social work education.

Gary P. Cournoyer, MSW, LICSW, is currently employed as an Administrator at Newport County Community Mental Health Center in the Children's Intensive Services Program. He previously worked for over 18 years in Rhode Island's Juvenile prison. Gary is a credentialed Pet Assisted Therapy Facilitator working with his rescued chocolate Labrador retriever, Cisco. With Cisco, Gary and his wife Anne share their home with two other rescue dogs: Shiloh, a 7-year-old Beagle and Daphne, a 2-year-old Beagle-Jack Russell mix.

Catherine A. Faver, PhD, LMSW, is Professor of Social Work at the University of Texas-Pan American. Her research focuses on animal abuse and family violence and on spirituality and social work.

Mary Montminy-Danna, LICSW, PhD, is Assistant Professor of Social Work at Salve Regina University in Newport, Rhode Island. She has held that appointment for the past 18 years. Her major responsibilities include teaching practice and policy courses and coordinating the field experience for junior and senior social work majors. She is currently the clinical consultant for the Women's Resource Center of Newport and Bristol Counties, Inc. Dr. Montminy-Danna is a trainer for the State of Rhode Island on the LINKS between animal cruelty and interpersonal violence. She has conducted research in this area and on children living with violence and school performance.

Judee E. Onyskiw, RN, PhD, is an educator and research advisor in the Faculty of Health and Community Studies at MacEwan College in Edmonton, Alberta. Prior to her current position, she was a Canada Research Chair in Family Violence and Health at the University of New Brunswick. Her research has primarily involved examining the impact of exposure to family violence on children's health, well-being, and social development and identifying factors that provide vulnerable children with some resilience.

Mary Lou Randour, PhD, is a psychologist who was a practicing clinician for 17 years. She received post-graduate training at the Cambridge Hospital at Harvard Medical School and the Washington Psychoanalytic Institute and holds the position of Adjunct Assistant Professor of Psychiatry at the Uniformed Services University of the Health Services. Dr. Randour offers training seminars to law enforcement and court personnel, mental health professionals, educators, animal control and humane society officers, and advocates for domestic violence victims and child protective service workers. The training seminars address the link between animal abuse and human violence as well as the assessment and treatment of animal abuse committed by children and adults. In addition to offering workshops and seminars, Dr. Randour identifies legislative and policy opportunities that address this important link and organizes efforts in support of them. She is the author of three handbooks: "A Common Bond: Maltreated Children and Animals in the Home" (forthcoming); *AniCare Child: An Assessment and Treatment Approach for Childhood Animal Abuse*; and second author of *The AniCare Model of Treatment for Animal Abuse*, which is designed for use with adults. Dr. Randour also is editor of one book and author of two; her latest book is titled *Animal Grace.*

Karen D. Schaefer, PhD, received her doctorate in counseling psychology from the University of Illinois at Urbana-Champaign. She is the training coordinator at New Mexico State University Counseling Center. In addition to training and supervision, her areas of professional interest include adult survivors of childhood abuse (physical, emotional, sexual, neglect) or trauma, grief and loss issues, offenders of abuse, animal abuse including offenders and victims who witnessed such abuse, the healing aspects of human-animal interactions and the provision of animal assisted therapy as an adjunct to psychotherapy.

Clarissa M. Uttley, MS, is a Behavioral Science doctoral student at the University of Rhode Island, where she received a Master's Degree. in Human Development and Family Studies. She is also a credentialed Pet Assisted Therapy Facilitator and works alongside her dog, Nina, at early childhood centers.

Preface

There was a trial in Florida involving an alleged murder for hire. A battered woman was accused, along with her son, of plotting to kill her husband, who had been murdered by a neighbor. The husband had brutalized her for a period of time as was documented by witnesses and her injuries. As an expert witness in the case, the senior author found it challenging to portray his brutality because of his disability. Called the 'Lobster Boy' in the carnival circles where he worked as an attraction, the husband's arms extended to just below the elbows only. Similarly, his legs ended just below the knees.

The jury seemed interested when he was depicted as beating and raping her. His driving at a high speed with her, family members, and the family dog in the car was described. He opened a car window and threw the dog out to its death. Immediately after hearing this, the jury as a whole emitted a groan that was heard across the courtroom. The woman was sobbing at the recollection. There was silence for a few minutes. The woman received a surprising light sentence, and some jury members felt that his behavior toward the dog was indicative of the depth of his violence.

Laws protecting animals are growing in many states across the country. According to the Humane Society of the United States, as of April 2006, 42 states have enacted felony-level penalties for certain acts of animal cruelty; 28 of these have occurred within the last 10 years. Other federal legislation includes such acts as the Animal Fighting Prohibition Enforcement Act, which establishes a felony-level penalty of up to three years of jail time for any interstate or foreign transport of animals for fighting purposes. This is part of a growing recognition of the important role that animals play in our lives.

[Haworth co-indexing entry note]: "Preface." Loring, Marti T., Robert Geffner, and Janessa March. Co-published simultaneously in *Journal of Emotional Abuse* (The Haworth Maltreatment & Trauma Press, an imprint of The Haworth Press) Vol. 7, No. 3, 2007, pp. xxi-xxiii; and: *Animal Abuse and Family Violence: Linkages, Research, and Implications for Professional Practice* (ed: Marti T. Loring, Robert Geffner, and Janessa Marsh) The Haworth Maltreatment & Trauma Press, an imprint of The Haworth Press, 2007, pp. xvii-xix. Single or multiple copies of this article are available for a fee from The Haworth Document Delivery Service [1-800-HAWORTH, 9:00 a.m. - 5:00 p.m. (EST). E-mail address: docdelivery@haworthpress.com].

In the mental health field, we have Frank Ascione to thank for our growing awareness of the significant role that animals play in the growth and development of children. His research has provided the foundation for understanding many dynamics of children and adults' maltreatment of animals, as well as their subsequent harm to humans. His ground-breaking work has provided us with a vision of why some battered women hesitate to seek safety in shelters. They will not leave their animals to a likely fate of injury at the hands of the batterer. Thus, coalitions have grown allowing women to go to shelters while leaving their animals in an equally safe place. Dr. Ascione's leadership in building coalitions has provided additional information and services, especially about the conjoined issues of cruelty to women and children and cruelty to animals. He has explored the relationship between animal violence and human violence. He reminds us of the invaluable work done by the American Humane Association, The Humane Society of the United States, and The Latham Foundation for the Promotion of Humane Education.

The following introduction is based on Dr. Ascione's book, *Children and Animals: Exploring the Roots of Kindness and Cruelty* (2004), as well as an interview conducted while he was working on his new international handbook on animals. The following articles by innovative authors are part of the culmination of the last 20 years during which greater awareness, research, and programs have developed in the area of our connections to animals and the dynamics and tragedy of their maltreatment.

There is a connection and love many humans share with their pets, many of whom are often considered an integral part of the family. Many people feel a love for animals and are moved by their helplessness in the face of violence. This deep love and loyalty has a universal quality that has caused some battered women to resist leaving a pet to enter a shelter, has caused some men and women to refuse to leave their flood-ravaged homes in New Orleans in the wake of Hurricane Katrina unless their pets could accompany them, and has caused some coerced people to obey an abuser's orders to commit an illegal act rather than risking harm to the pet who is being threatened.

The authors and editors invite readers to appreciate the contributions of those who historically have given us the foundation for our continued quest and to learn from the innovative research and writing here that will enrich our knowledge. We regret any discomfort experienced after reading about animal maltreatment. We appreciate our connections with animals and deeply regret the tragic maltreatment some humans and animals suffer at the hands of other humans. We applaud creative programs, some to be described, that engender prevention of cruelty to animals and nonviolence toward humans.

Marti T. Loring
Robert Geffner
Janessa Marsh

Introduction:
Animal Abuse and Family Violence

Marti T. Loring
Janessa Marsh
Robert Geffner

SUMMARY. The present collection of articles attempts to shrink the literature gap that currently exists in the areas of animal abuse and its relation to family violence. This introductory chapter outlines the historical issues of animal cruelty, based specifically on an interview with Frank Ascione, a pioneer in exploring the issue of abuse of animals and the reasons for its occurrence. Definitions of animal maltreatment, ramifications of its commission, and future directions for research and practice are discussed. A detailed outline for the present volume is also provided, painting a clear picture of the need for this and future books on the issues. doi:10.1300/J135v07n03_01 *[Article copies available for a fee from The Haworth Document Delivery Service: 1-800-HAWORTH. E-mail address: <docdelivery@haworthpress.com> Website: <http://www.HaworthPress.com> © 2007 by The Haworth Press. All rights reserved.]*

KEYWORDS. Animal cruelty, family violence, pet abuse, research, professional practice

---

Address correspondence to: Marti T. Loring, PhD, LCSW (E-mail: mloring@earthlink.net).

[Haworth co-indexing entry note]: "Introduction: Animal Abuse and Family Violence." Loring, Marti T., Janessa Marsh, and Robert Geffner. Co-published simultaneously in *Journal of Emotional Abuse* (The Haworth Maltreatment & Trauma Press, an imprint of The Haworth Press) Vol. 7, No. 3, 2007, pp. 1-6; and: *Animal Abuse and Family Violence: Linkages, Research, and Implications for Professional Practice* (ed: Marti T. Loring, Robert Geffner, and Janessa Marsh) The Haworth Maltreatment & Trauma Press, an imprint of The Haworth Press, 2007, pp. 1-6. Single or multiple copies of this article are available for a fee from The Haworth Document Delivery Service [1-800-HAWORTH, 9:00 a.m. - 5:00 p.m. (EST). E-mail address: docdelivery@haworthpress.com].

THE ORIGINS OF THE ISSUES:
CONTRIBUTIONS OF FRANK ASCIONE

In his search for a definition of animal abuse, Frank Ascione, a pioneer in exploring the relationship between humans and animals, has suggested that animal abuse be defined as "socially unacceptable behavior that intentionally causes unnecessary pain, suffering, or distress to and/or the death of an animal" (Ascione, 1993, p. 228). According to Ascione, challenges with defining and measuring animal abuse have contributed to its being "dormant for long" (p. 30). There has been an absence of standardized reporting and of recording such abuse. Efforts over the last two decades have included studies to measure the presence and types of animal abuse. These goals have sometimes been joint efforts by researchers and agencies serving animals. Indeed, the rediscovery of the relationship between animal and human welfare has brought greater attention to the connection between harm to animals and violence toward children and adults.

As Ascione indicated in an interview with the authors, early in his graduate studies he wondered why there was so little attention paid to what he considered an important area: the role of animals in the development of children (personal communication, April 2, 2007). He would later find himself in the forefront of advocacy, research, writing, and speaking about animal cruelty, as his most current book suggests, *Children and Animals: Exploring the Roots of Kindness and Cruelty* (2004). In his book, Ascione depicts the mutual love and caring between pets and their families. He explores the ways in which children's growth and development are impacted by having an animal in the home, sharing in caretaking responsibilities for the pet, and learning gentleness with which a pet should be treated. There is an exploration of how parents can teach this gentleness while modeling it themselves in the way they are treating not only the pet, but their children and each other as well.

In the interview with Ascione, he acknowledged that abused women and children have actually been our teachers; they have related to us the deep meaning that animals have to them and the profound pain experienced when their pets are threatened and harmed. These victims have brought our attention back to other victims without a voice: the animals that are also considered by many as family members. Efforts to serve battered women and children in shelters have, more and more, included assisting with the safe care of their pets. Some had refused to enter shelters when it meant leaving the pet to probable harm and even possible death at the hands of an abuser.

The history and current contributions of such agencies as the American Humane Association and The Humane Society of the United States have been profound in direct service to animals, education about the link between cruelty of animals and violence to people, and research efforts. In fact, when Ascione was struggling to have time from his teaching responsibilities to write his recent book (2004), not only did the Kenneth A. Scott Charitable Trust Foundation for the Promotion of Humane Education step forward to offer financial support, but American Humane shared as well in financially supporting this important effort. The royalties from the book go to the American Humane Association.

Why would someone harm or kill an animal, cause it suffering or distress? Acknowledging the contributions of Kellert and Felthous (1985) in the area of categorizing animal maltreatment, Ascione describes adult motivation for animal abuse: control or discipline, retaliation against a person, to satisfy a prejudice toward certain species or breeds of animals, enhancing person aggressiveness, and sadism (Ascione, 2005). For children's motivation to abuse animals, he explores peer reinforcement, attempts to modify their mood, incidents where the children are enticed, coerced or forced to abuse animals, attachment to an animal (rather than letting someone abuse it), identification with the aggressor, imitating adult treatment of pets and other animals, to using an animal as an implement of self-injury, posttraumatic play, monetary gain, or rehearsal for interpersonal violence.

Another historical development in relation to animal abuse is the growing recognition of the relationship between animal maltreatment and empathy, or the lack thereof. That is, among those who abuse animals with so little empathy for their discomfort or the anguish of their human owners, there are many people who also abuse partners or children. A part of the historical development of studying animal abuse has included exploring prison populations for histories of violence to humans and animals. In fact, there is growing recognition that the lack of empathy in youthful animal abusers may well predict later violence to humans. Thus, programs enhancing empathy and gentleness have become important applications of the knowledge we are learning about animal maltreatment.

Ascione hopes for further studies and program development in the area of animal abuse. For example, he noted that sexual abuse of animals has not received a great deal of attention (2005). In regard to policy, he hopes that humane societies and veterinarians will collect data regarding animal abuse and track these over time, perhaps some day contributing it to a national data bank. Longitudinal research and the development of more consistent assessments would also aid in filling the information void, leading to better prevention and intervention efforts.

THE PRESENT VOLUME

The present collection of articles attempts to shrink the literature gap that currently exists in the areas of animal abuse and its relation to family violence. In the opening article of this collection, Onyskiw provides a concise overview of empirical literature in existence relating to family violence and its linkages to cruelty to family pets. As noted in the article, as well as by Ascione, while modest attention has been paid to this link in scholarly literature, mainstream media has yet to tackle this growing issue. Implications for professionals with regard to intervention and prevention efforts are also discussed, providing a solid framework and background for the rest of this volume.

The next article by Schaefer outlines in-depth the short- and long-term effects of experiencing animal abuse and the impact this has on victims. She proposes that witnessing, being threatened with or being forced to commit animal abuse is an additional form of maltreatment that could provoke short- and long-term effects for the victim, especially when this form of abuse is coupled with other types of abuse in the home (e.g., intimate partner violence, physical and/or emotional abuse). The article includes case examples of clients experiencing multiple forms of abuse, including the witnessing or commission of animal abuse, and the ramifications of these experiences are discussed along with recommendations for addressing these types of traumas.

In the next two articles, new empirical research not previously explored with regard to animal abuse is provided. In the article by Faver and Cavazos, the authors introduce new findings from a survey of women, primarily Hispanic, who sought help from a domestic violence shelter near the U.S.-Mexico border. The study contributes significant new findings regarding the Hispanic population and pet abuse, specifically that pet abuse is a component of intimate partner violence in this community.

The study by Montminy-Danna investigates the prevalence of animal cruelty disclosure in child welfare cases. In a survey of child welfare workers, findings suggest that almost one-quarter of cases include disclosures of animal abuse; unfortunately, there is no standard protocol in place for addressing these incidents. Qualitative findings provide expanded information (e.g., types of abuse, perpetrators of cruelty), and recommendations from those surveyed are discussed.

As many of the articles note, there are no consistent or mandated reporting or collection standards dealing with animal cruelty, and thus valuable information is continually lost. Randour's article explores policy implications at the state and federal levels to promote both the collection of data and communication among agencies; offered are proposals for including questions regarding animal cruelty into federal databases. She also reviews professional standards for the mental health profession, providing suggestions for including animal cruelty as an important component for assessment and treatment in the areas of education and training for mental health professionals.

The final article provides a positive outlook to the sobering issues explored in this volume. Cisco's Kids, a behavioral intervention program utilizing pet assisted therapy, has seen over 50 incarcerated youth successfully complete the curriculum. Cournoyer, the lead author and owner of the therapy pet Cisco, discusses the qualitative data gathered over two and a half years since the program's inception. A brief history of Pet-Assisted Therapy is given, illustrating that utilizing the human-animal bond in a positive way can have enormous rewards.

As Ascione commented in his interview, the more we learn about a certain topic, the more we realize how much we do not know about that area. In terms of the topic of animal cruelty, we hope this collection of articles fills a void not previously investigated. The articles aim to provide new insights, spur new research, and change the way animal cruelty is viewed and dealt with in our families and our communities.

AUTHOR NOTE

Marti T. Loring, PhD, LCSW, is a social worker and sociologist in Atlanta, Georgia. She is director of the Center for Mental Health and Human Development; and the Emotional Abuse Institute. Dr. Loring's expertise is in the areas of abuse and trauma. She has taught in several universities and conducted training seminars. She has written several articles published in professional journals and two books, including *Emotional Abuse*. An evaluator in court cases, Dr. Loring has testified across the country in cases including issues of animal abuse. Some of her research has involved the role of pet abuse in family violence; in particular, animal abuse as a means of coercion when battered women are forced into illegal acts.

Janessa Marsh, MA, is Assistant Editor for the *Journal of Aggression, Maltreatment & Trauma*, the *Journal of Child Sexual Abuse*, the *Journal of Emotional Abuse*, and the new *Journal of Child and Adolescent Trauma* and is on staff at the Institute on Violence, Abuse and Trauma at Alliant International University in San Diego, CA. Ms.

Marsh received her Master's Degree in Industrial-Organizational Psychology from the California School of Organizational Studies at Alliant International University and her undergraduate degree from Louisiana State University.

Robert Geffner, PhD, ABPP, ABPN, is Founder and President of the Family Violence and Sexual Assault Institute in San Diego, CA; President of Alliant International University's Institute on Violence, Abuse and Trauma; Acting Director of Alliant's Center of Forensic Studies; Clinical Research Professor of Psychology at the California School of Professional Psychology, Alliant International University; Licensed Psychologist and Licensed Marriage & Family Therapist in California and Texas; Editor-in-Chief of Haworth's Maltreatment and Trauma Press, which also includes being the Editor of three internationally disseminated journals (*Journal of Child Sexual Abuse* and *Journal of Aggression, Maltreatment & Trauma,* and co-editor of *Journal of Emotional Abuse*); and former clinical director of a large private practice mental health clinic in East Texas for over 15 years. He has a Diplomate in Clinical Neuropsychology and one in Family Psychology. He served as an adjunct faculty member for the National Judicial College for 10 years, and was a former Professor of Psychology at the University of Texas at Tyler for 16 years. He has also been a researcher and consultant during the past 25 years. Publications include recent treatment manuals, edited books concerning family violence and child maltreatment, one book in press, and numerous book chapters, journal articles and research papers concerning family violence, sexual assault, child abuse, family and child psychology, custody issues, forensic psychology, neuropsychology and diagnostic assessment. He has also served on several national and state committees dealing with various aspects of family psychology, family violence, child abuse, and family law. He has presented over 450 keynote addresses, plenaries, workshops, and seminars at international, national, regional, and state conferences or meetings.

REFERENCES

Ascione, F. R. (1993). Children who are cruel to animals: A review of research and implications for developmental psychopathology. *Anthrozoos*, *6*, 226-247.

Ascione, F. R. (2005). *Children and animals: Exploring the roots of kindness and cruelty*. West Lafayette, IN: Purdue University Press.

Kellert, S. R., & Felthous, A. R. (1985). Childhood cruelty toward animals among criminals and noncriminals. *Human Relations*, *38*, 1113-1129.

doi:10.1300/J135v07n03_01

THE RELATIONSHIP AND IMPACT
OF ANIMAL CRUELTY
IN FAMILY VIOLENCE

The Link Between Family Violence
and Cruelty to Family Pets

Judee E. Onyskiw

SUMMARY. Family violence remains a prevalent social problem cross-ing racial, geographic, social, and economic boundaries (World Health Organization, 2002). Different forms of family violence often exist in the same households. In the 1980s, researchers observed a connection be-tween acts of animal cruelty and family violence. Since then other re-searchers have corroborated their findings. Despite these articles appearing in the scholarly literature, there has been relatively little atten-tion given to this issue in mainstream literature on family violence and lit-tle evidence that this information has been used to inform prevention or intervention efforts. This article summarizes the empirical evidence on the link between family violence and cruelty to family pets and discusses the

Address correspondence to: Judee E. Onyskiw, Faculty of Health and Community Studies, MacEwan College, Edmonton, Alberta, Canada, T5J 4S2 (E-mail: onyskiwj2@macewan.ca).

[Haworth co-indexing entry note]: "The Link Between Family Violence and Cruelty to Family Pets." Onyskiw, Judee E. Co-published simultaneously in *Journal of Emotional Abuse* (The Haworth Maltreatment & Trauma Press, an imprint of The Haworth Press) Vol. 7, No. 3, 2007, pp. 7-30; and: *Animal Abuse and Family Violence: Linkages, Research, and Implications for Professional Practice* (ed: Marti T. Loring, Robert Geffner, and Janessa Marsh) The Haworth Maltreatment & Trauma Press, an imprint of The Haworth Press, 2007, pp. 7-30. Single or multiple copies of this article are available for a fee from The Haworth Document Delivery Service [1-800-HAWORTH, 9:00 a.m. - 5:00 p.m. (EST). E-mail address: docdelivery@ haworthpress.com].

implications of these connections for professionals who work with women, children, families, or animals. doi:10.1300/J135v07n03_02 *[Article copies available for a fee from The Haworth Document Delivery Service: 1-800-HAWORTH. E-mail address: <docdelivery@haworthpress.com> Website: <http://www.HaworthPress.com> © 2007 by The Haworth Press. All rights reserved.]*

KEYWORDS. Family violence, woman abuse, pet abuse, links, child abuse, domestic violence, animal cruelty, connections

Despite notable efforts to eliminate violence in families, family violence remains a pressing and prevalent social problem. Violence occurs at every level of society crossing racial, geographic, social, and economic boundaries (World Health Organization, 2002). Women are injured or humiliated by violent partners, children are abused or neglected by parents or older siblings, and the elderly are maltreated or economically deprived by adult children or grandchildren. Violence pervades families in our society. Although women are violent toward their male partners, and violence occurs between partners of the same gender, in the majority of cases of partner violence, women are victimized by men (Johnson, 1996; United States Department of Justice, 2005). In population-based surveys conducted in the United States (U.S.) and in Canada, 25 to 30% of women report being physically abused by an intimate partner at some point in their lives (Johnson, 1996; Jones et al., 1999; Tjaden & Thoennes, 2000). Every year, an estimated 3 to 10 million American children and 1 to 2 million Canadian children are exposed to violence in their own homes. Children are exposed to a range of abusive behavior, from hearing insults and name-calling to acts of extreme aggression using weapons, including witnessing murder (Lewandowski, McFarlane, Campbell, Gary, & Barenski, 2004).

Children are also the direct victims of violence. In the United States, 11% of all violent crimes occurring within families are committed by parents against their children (U.S. Department of Justice, 2005). Children and youth are 10 times more likely to be victims of violence than to be arrested for violent crimes. In Canada, children account for about 25% of all victims of physical assault, and 61% of sexual assault cases (Statistics Canada, 2005). Of those assaults that are family related, 70% of the physical assaults and 40% of the sexual assaults are perpetrated by parents (Statistics Canada, 2005). Children are far more likely to be abused by family members than strangers.

Although statistics on woman abuse and child abuse are collected and presented separately, these different forms of family violence do not always exist independently of one another. Most often, one form of violence in the home is an indicator that other family members are at risk. The link between woman abuse and child abuse has long been recognized (Anaya, 2004; Appel & Holden, 1998; Edelson, 1999; Folsom, Christensen, Avery, & Moore, 2003; Lee, Kotch, & Cox, 2004; McKay, 1994; Osofsky, 2003; Ross, 1996; Tajima, 2000). In homes where women are abused, children are more likely to be abused. Following a review of studies assessing the overlap between woman abuse and child abuse, Appel and Holden (1998) found that the percentage ranged from 20% to 100% with a median rate of 40% reported in clinical samples of abused women or children. Children are at risk for all types of abuse, including physical, sexual, emotional abuse and neglect perpetrated by mothers, fathers, or both parents.

Several researchers have observed that there is also a connection between acts of animal cruelty and different forms of violence in families. Over 20 years ago, a British researcher published a scholarly paper documenting the connection between animal cruelty and the physical abuse of children (Hutton, 1983). At the same time, researchers in the United States noted that a large percentage of families referred to child protective services for child maltreatment showed a breakdown in their capacity to care for their pets. They suggested the need to systematically study the relationship between the treatment of animals and humans (DeViney, Dickert, & Lockwood, 1983). More recently, Flynn (1999) published an article eloquently documenting the reasons that family professionals needed to pay serious attention to violence toward animals while Beirne (2002) urged criminologists to include investigating the causes of animal abuse in their research agenda. Despite these articles appearing in the scholarly literature, there has been relatively little attention given to this issue in mainstream literature on family violence and little evidence that this information has been used to inform prevention or intervention efforts. The purpose of this article is to review research on the link between family violence and cruelty to family pets. The objectives of the review are to: (1) summarize empirical evidence, (2) raise awareness of the connections between family violence and cruelty to family pets, and (3) discuss the implications of these connections for professionals who work with women, children, families, and/or animals.

DEFINITIONS OF ABUSE

Abuse in humans has been difficult to define despite decades of scholarly discussion and debate (Dobash & Dobash, 1992; DeKeseredy, 2000; Gelles, 2000a; Onyskiw, 2005; Saltzmann, Fanslow, McMahon, & Shelley, 1999). For the purposes of this article, abuse refers to physical, sexual, psychological or emotional mistreatment, and other controlling tactics such as economic or spiritual deprivation against an intimate partner (including married, cohabiting, or dating, current or estranged intimate partner) by the other partner. Abuse begins in subtle forms that are often difficult to detect. There is usually an insidious pattern of abuse already occurring when violence happens (Campbell, 2000). Abuse is best conceptualized as a *pattern of behavior and experiences* used to achieve domination and control in the relationship (Campbell, 2000; Dobash & Dobash, 1979, 1992; Gordon, 2000; Yllo, 1993).

Abuse and neglect in relation to children also has been difficult to define. Federal legislation, specifically the Child Abuse Prevention and Treatment Act of 1974, and its amendments, defines child abuse and neglect broadly as any recent act or failure to act resulting in imminent risk of serious harm, death, serious physical or emotional harm, sexual abuse, or exploitation of a child (a person under the age of 18) by a parent or caretaker who is responsible for the child's welfare. Child abuse is frequently divided into four categories (i.e., physical abuse, sexual abuse, emotional abuse and neglect). For some time, children's exposure to domestic violence has been recognized as harmful to children and a form of emotional abuse. In the United States, several states (i.e., Alaska, Georgia, Minnesota, and Utah) include witnessing domestic violence in child abuse legislation (Kantor & Little, 2003; Zink Kamine, Sill, Field, & Putman, 2004). The state of Utah has legislation that makes the commission of a domestic assault in the presence of a child at least two or more times chargeable as a misdemeanor (Zink et al., 2004). In Canada, witnessing domestic violence is included in legislation for child abuse in 6 of the 10 provinces (i.e., Alberta, Saskatchewan, Prince Edward Island, New Brunswick, Nova Scotia, and Newfoundland; Echlin & Marshall, 1995). Nevertheless, the issue of including exposure to domestic violence in child abuse legislation remains contentious. There has been inconsistent use of these alternatives and skepticism about whether they are always in the best interests of the child or the mother (see Echlin & Marshall, 1995; Kantor & Little, 2003 for a discussion).

Similar to abuse in humans, animal abuse also has been difficult to define (Agnew, 1998). Drawing on Ascione (1993), a researcher whose program of research has focused on the link between human and animal abuse, abuse is broadly defined as socially unacceptable behavior that intentionally causes unnecessary pain, suffering, or distress to and/or death of an animal (p. 228). This definition includes physical abuse and neglect, including acts of commission and omission, and sexual abuse involving bestiality. While physical harm is the easiest form of abuse to recognize, neglect is the most prevalent, occurring in almost 90% of all cases of animal abuse (Solot, 1997). The terms animal abuse and cruelty to animals are used interchangeably.

A SUMMARY OF EMPIRICAL EVIDENCE

In the 1980s, in work that was pioneering at the time, researchers in Britain noted the link between child abuse and cruelty to animals. Hutton (1983) examined the files of 23 families in a British community brought to the attention of the Royal Society for the Prevention of Cruelty to Animals (RSPCA). He found that 82% of the families were known to local social service agencies as having children at risk for signs of neglect and physical abuse, while 61% of the families were known to probation services.

At the same time, DeViney and her colleagues (1983) investigated the treatment of animals in 53 families meeting state criteria in New Jersey for substantiated child abuse and neglect. Using home observations, 60% of the families were identified as having met at least one of the criteria for pet abuse according to those established by Leavitt (1978 cited in DeViney et al., 1983). A wide range of abuse was reported from causing pain and suffering to the death of the animal. The most common pattern of abuse occurred when an abusive parent or stepparent targeted one or more children, as well as a pet, and used violence against the pet to intimidate or control the child. Animal abuse was significantly higher (88%) in families where children had been physically abused than in families that emotionally or sexually abused or neglected their children (34%; DeViney et al., 1983). In the majority of abusive incidents, the parents were responsible; however, children were reported to hit, kick, pester or annoy pets in 26% of the families. DeViney and her colleagues (1983) concluded that there were parallels between the treatment of children and the treatment of pets in child abusing families, and that the capacity to care for a pet may signal other forms of abuse and neglect in the family. While these studies involved small numbers and lacked control groups, they did suggest a connection between child abuse and animal abuse in families.

Ascione, Weber, and Wood (1997a) conducted one of the first studies to examine pet abuse in the lives of abused women. They surveyed 101 women in shelters for abused women in Utah and compared their responses to a community sample of 60 women who were not abused.

All women owned pets. Compared to women in the community group, the shelter women were three times more likely to report that their partners had threatened to harm their pets (52% versus 16.7%), and 15 times more likely to report that their partners had actually harmed or killed their pets (54% versus 3.5%). In the majority of cases, the shelter women reported that there had been multiple incidents of abusing pets. Ascione, Weber, and Wood (1997b) also conducted a national survey of shelters in the United States. They surveyed the largest shelter in 49 states and the District of Columbia. Shelters were selected if they provided overnight facilities and programs or services for children. Ninety-six percent of the shelters responded. Of these shelters, 85.4% reported that women using their services spoke about incidents of abuse of their family pets. In another study, 38 women seeking shelter at a safe house voluntarily completed surveys about pet ownership (Ascione, 1998). Of these women, 71% reported that their partners had threatened or actually harmed or killed one or more of their pets.

Other researchers reported high rates of pet abuse in samples of women seeking refuge from abuse. In a survey of over 100 battered women in shelters, Flynn (2000a) found that almost half of the women with pets reported that their male partners had threatened, hurt, or killed their companion animals. Quinlisk (1999) found that 68% of women in shelters reported that their pets had been abused. In 88% of the incidents, women had witnessed the abuse. Almost 50% of the women in Faver and Strand's (2003a) study reported that their partner had threatened to harm their pet and 46% had actually harmed their pet. A similar study to assess the prevalence of pet abuse in homes experiencing domestic violence was conducted by the Ontario Society for the Prevention of Cruelty to Animals in Canada. They interviewed over 100 women at 21 battered women's shelters across the province and found that 44% of battered women reported that their partner had abused or killed family pets.

The strongest evidence of a connection between animal abuse and family violence, however, comes from a recent case-control study of intimate partner homicide conducted in 11 cities across the United States. Walton-Moss, Manganello, Frye, and Campbell (2005) found that pet abuse was a strong risk factor for intimate partner violence. The sample consisted of women who had survived an attempted homicide and proxies for women who were murdered by their intimate partners. Proxies were usually the victim's mother, sister, or a friend and were used so that researchers could obtain data on the murdered women. Findings showed that compared to non-abused women, women who reported that their partners had abused a pet were 7.6 times more likely to be abused. In fact, pet abuse was a stronger risk factor for abuse than having fair or poor mental health (Adjusted Odds Ratio [AOR] = 6.6), having problems with drinking (AOR = 2.8) or drugs (AOR = 1.9), or not completing high school (AOR = 2.1; Walton-Moss et al., 2005). These latter factors are generally accepted as being related to an increased risk for abuse. The association between partner violence and animal abuse is not confined to heterosexual relationships. Renzelli (1992) discovered that 38% of lesbian partners had harmed family pets.

In violent families, children are often exposed to violence between their parents, most often violence directed at their mothers. Children also are exposed to abuse of their family pet. Almost half of the children in one study of women in shelters witnessed their pets being abused compared to less than 4% of the community sample (Ascione et al., 1997a). In their national survey of shelters, Ascione and his colleagues (1997b) found that children of women in safe-houses were 20 times more likely to have witnessed pet abuse than community children. Over 64% of shelter women in McIntosh's (2001) study and 76% of the women in Quinlisk's (1999) study reported that children witnessed their pets' abuse.

WHY PETS IN VIOLENT FAMILIES ARE TARGETED

The majority of households in the United States have pets (American Veterinary Association, 1997). Many people consider their pets to be members of the family (Albert & Bulcroft, 1988) and are emotionally attached to them (Flynn, 2000a, 2000b). They buy their pets special treats, talk to them in a conversational style, take them on holidays, give them presents on special occasions, allow their pets to sleep in their beds, and grieve their loss when they die (Carmack, 1985). In essence, people treat their pets like valued family members. Unfortunately, their status as family members, like other members of families (children, adults, and seniors) puts them at risk for abuse.

Women who are abused, like other women in the general population, report a strong emotional attachment to their pets. Abused women may be even more emotionally attached to their pets than individuals who live violence-free lives because of the chaos and emotional trauma and the isolation they experience. Pets are an important source of support, a companion for many women. When women are isolated, they may substitute pets for human interaction in their lives (Flynn, 2000a; 2000b).

Pets may be an especially important support for women without children. Women without children in Flynn's study (2000a) were almost twice as likely as women with children to report that their pets were an important source of emotional support. The stronger the emotional attachment to the pet, the more likely the pet was harmed. Women without children more frequently reported that their pets had been threatened or harmed than women with children. Women with both children and pets whose pets were abused were more likely to report their children had also been abused.

Abusers recognize the special relationship that victims have with their pets and use this to their advantage. A feminist explanation points out that power, domination, and control underlies all forms of violence against women (Counts, Brown, & Campbell, 1999; Dobash & Dobash, 1979; Walker, 1979; Yllo, 1993). Typically, abusers attempt to dominate and control by engaging in actions that threaten or harm a women's physical or emotional well-being (Campbell, 2000). Women's subordination is secured when they become fearful of future abuse and alter their behavior to avoid negative reprisals from their abusive partner (Stark & Flitcraft, 1996). By abusing or threatening to harm the pet, the perpetrator exerts his domination and control and eliminates the woman's source of comfort. Perpetrators harm or threaten to harm animals to intimidate, frighten, terrorize, control, and silence their victims allowing the abuse to continue (Adams, 1998; Becker & French, 2004; Faver & Strand, 2003b; Kogan, McConnell, Schoenfeld-Tacher, & Jansen-Lock, 2004). Women are forced into abusive situations or forced into remaining silent about the abuse because they fear that their cherished pet will be hurt. Abusing pets are a powerful means of control and intimidation. When people care deeply about their pets, it is terrorizing to have someone threaten or hurt them.

By abusing the pet, or merely threatening abuse, the perpetrator sends a strong message warning the women that they may be next (Suthers-McCabe, 2005). Threats or actual harm to pets gives the perpetrator control over the victim even when the victim is not in their presence. It is a powerful and poignant form of emotional blackmail that gives the perpetrator power at all times and gains the victim's cooperation and submission. The message is so powerful that some women do not leave violent partners because they are afraid that their partner will harm or kill their pet once they leave the home. Women also stay because it is difficult to find accommodation where they can take their pets. Thus, many women remain in abusive relationships.

Some researchers have noted that physical abuse may lessen as these emotionally abusive tactics escalate (Jacobson & Gottman, 1998). Other researchers found the opposite. Ascione and his associates (1997a) noted that physical abuse actually escalated when perpetrators threaten to harm pets and abusers who threatened or harmed pets also more severely physically abused their partners.

Abusing family pets is also an effective method to coerce and control children, since pets are also an integral part of children's lives (Ascione et al., 1997b). In the context of violence against their mothers, cruelty to family pets may be used to coerce, control, or intimidate children, to obtain their silence about the abuse or to ensure their cooperation. Children's exposure to the abuse of their mothers or their pets constitutes a form of emotional abuse known as terrorizing (Ascione, 1998; Ascione et al., 1997a). In the context of child sexual abuse, threats of abuse or harming pets are used to gain control over the child, ensuring their silence and submission. Children are forced to choose between their victimization and their pet's survival (Adams, 1998).

While woman and children regard their pets as family members, the notion of pets as family members contrasts sharply with the perspective taken by most abusers. Pets may be subjected to abuse because their abusers, at least in part, consider them property. Carlisle-Frank, Frank, and Nielsen (2004) recently conducted a survey of women in shelters to determine the batterer's attitudes, perceptions, and behaviors toward pets. Seventy percent of the women reported that their batterers viewed their pets as property. According to their reports, the less positive the abuser's attitude toward the family pet, the more likely the pet was abused. There was a distinct difference between the attitudes and behaviors of batterers who did and did not abuse their pets. Batterers who had more favorable attitudes toward their family pets did not abuse them. Ninety percent of pet abusers were reported to never show their pets affection, while 57% of pet non-abusers showed affection at least occasionally. There was also a difference between pet abusers and non-abusers in how they spoke to their pets. Ninety-five percent of pet abusers were reported to speak only using commands, whereas 79% of non-abusers were reported to speak using a conversational style (Carlisle-Frank et al., 2004).

A social-psychological explanation for animal abuse is the notion that the perceived benefits outweigh the costs for the person who abuses animals (Agnew, 1998). The costs of most forms of animal abuse are low. There are few deterrents in society to prevent animal abuse. Abuse occurs in the privacy of homes, easily hidden from public view. Many cases go unreported–some for a long time–and are only discovered when living conditions are deplorable (Crook, 2005). There are few formal sanctions for abuse; they are rarely implemented when they do exist. When they are imposed, they typically are not serious. Advocates point out that people who are charged with abusing animals are not subjected to penalties that are harsh enough to act as a deterrent. Cruelty to animals is not taken as seriously as other crimes, or as seriously as it ought to be taken. Society may not view animal abuse as important as other forms of abuse. This may, in part, reflect animals' low status in society and the fact that they are viewed as private property (Agnew, 1998; Favre & Tsang, 1993). In Canada, there are some proposed amendments to the Criminal Code to classify animal cruelty as a criminal offense instead of a property offense. The amendments would improve the ability to prosecute offenders and would provide harsher penalties for offenses (Crook, 2005). Though laws will change when these amendments are passed, they need to be enforced to compel change in public conduct.

WHY WE HAVE BEEN SLOW TO RECOGNIZE THE LINK

One reason that we have been slow to recognize the link between different forms of violence in families may be a function of how society recognized the problem of abuse and responded to this issue. Western society has addressed the issue by developing separate organizations for women, children, elderly people, and animals. Over time, these organizations have evolved into very distinct entities.

Historically, society first recognized the need to protect animals from abuse and abandonment. In 1824, the Royal Society for the Prevention of Cruelty to Animals (RSPCA) was formed in Britain (Favre & Tsang, 1993). Similar organizations were formed in the United States in 1865 and in Canada in 1869. Organized efforts to protect children developed as an outgrowth of this humane work for animals. The Society for the Prevention of Cruelty to Children was formed in 1875 after the New York Society for the Prevention of Cruelty to Animals (SPCA) apprehended a little girl from her abusive home (Bremner, 1970; Cole, 1993; Zilney & Zilney, 2005). Mary Ellen Wilson had been routinely beaten, starved, and imprisoned by her adopted parents. Although her neighbors were outraged, no formal organization existed at the time to protect children. In desperation, they contacted the SPCA. The founder, Henry Bergh, together with an attorney, was able to remove Mary Ellen from her parents' home using laws created to protect animals. Subsequently, a formal organization was developed to protect children.

The anti-child abuse movement, however, lost visibility until the mid-twentieth century when it was brought to national attention by a pediatrician. Henry Kempe described child abuse as a clinical condition with physical symptoms and named it the "battered child syndrome" (Kempe, Silverman, Steele, Droemueller, & Silver, 1962). In spite of the considerable attention that Kempe drew from the media and the scholarly community, it was still another decade before woman abuse was recognized. Similar to child maltreatment, violence against women also had existed for centuries and had been sanctioned by society and deeply entrenched in cultural, legal, political, and religious traditions and institutions (Code, 1993; Dobash & Dobash, 1979). All family members were viewed as the property of the head of the household. It was the responsibility of men, as heads of the household, to punish and discipline their wives and children.

In the 1960s, the women's movement increased public awareness about violence against women. Social advocates called attention to the fact that women were being abused and that the family was in fact a violent institution. Their efforts led to a serious examination of the family and its structure to understand the nature of abuse and transformed a problem that had been virtually ignored to one that demanded professional, public, and policy attention (Yllo, 1993). Efforts were organized by grassroots organizations to provide safe refuge for women and their children fleeing abuse. Over time, advocates made significant efforts to develop badly needed programs and services for abused women (Yllo, 1993).

By the late twentieth century, separate organizations had developed to respond to the needs of abused animals, women, children, and even the elderly in our society. Separate advocacy groups exist, each championing their own cause. Different forms of family violence, for the most part, have been treated by different organizations despite knowledge that violence occurs among members of the same family. The development of different organizations may have obscured the fact that these various forms of violence do not occur independently of one another. Multiple forms of abuse often occur in the same household. Further, the development of distinct service delivery systems to respond to these various forms of abuse (animal abuse, child abuse, woman abuse, and elder abuse) means that these separate systems often compete for scarce resources, a factor which only serves to intensify separate agendas. With this increasing specialization and diversification, the problem of violence in families has become compartmentalized. Gelles (2000b) eloquently termed this compartmentalization into separate issues and sub-issues the "balkanization" of family violence and points out that there are deficiencies of this perspective (p. 298). These different organizations operate independently to prevent, detect, and treat their particular form of family violence, each operating with good intentions in their own specific area of concern (Gelles, 2000b). It is not surprising that policy makers, practitioners, and service providers frequently fail to recognize the direct and important connections among the different forms of violence in society to the detriment of families experiencing multiple forms of abuse.

It is not only organizations and policy makers who have a compartmentalized approach. Researchers who study these various forms of violence also tend to focus their efforts on one form of abuse, in one particular population, to the exclusion of other forms of abuse affecting other family members. Efforts may be focused on the abuse of women, children, or the elderly or even one particular subgroup of these populations, such as women who are sexually abused or children exposed to woman abuse. Researchers often present their work at conferences that specialize in a specific type of abuse (e.g., child abuse and neglect, violence against women) and publish their work in speciality journals. Thus, it is not surprising that over time the link between different forms of abuse has become obscured and forgotten.

Consequently, despite knowledge of the link between different forms of violence in families and cruelty toward animals, the integration of services for victims of family violence such as social services, child welfare, law enforcement and the judicial system has not occurred (Osofsky, 2003). Several scholars stress the need for various social service agencies as well as grassroots organizations to work together for mutual benefit (Ascione, 1993; Boat, 1995; Flynn, 2000c). A collaborative approach that addresses violence in all of its forms, including violence against animals, may help promote efforts to achieve a more humane and less violent society for all humans and animals.

WHY WE NEED TO ADDRESS CRUELTY TO ANIMALS WITHIN FAMILIES

There are compelling reasons for society to address cruelty to animals within families (Flynn, 2000c). In their own right, animals deserve humane treatment. Moral philosophers, social and feminist theorists have argued that animals deserve consideration in their own right (Agnew, 1998). Animal abuse is a disturbing, antisocial, and illegal behavior and a sign of serious psychopathology (Ascione, 1998). While animal abuse is an important phenomenon in its own right, it is also critical to address this issue because of its co-occurrence with other forms of violence in families. The treatment of animals is inextricably linked to the abuse of humans and may be an indicator that others are at risk in the family (Solot, 1997).

Addressing cruelty to animals may eliminate or at least alleviate a significant barrier for women wanting to leave an abusive situation. Women often delay going to a shelter because they are worried about their pets, putting themselves and their children at increased risk of harm. Almost one-quarter of the women in Ascione's (1997a) study delayed going to a shelter out of concern for their pets, while Carlisle-Frank and associates (2004) found 48% of victims delayed seeking shelter out of concern for their pets. In repeated cases of pet abuse, 65% of victims delayed seeking shelter while 25% of victims returned to the abuser out of concern for their pet.

Women are not only concerned about companion animals. Animal abuse against farm animals is a significant issue for women living in rural farming communities. In recent work, Doherty and Hornosty (2004) noted that rural women delayed seeking shelter because they were worried about the safety of farm animals. Women were worried about the animals' well being because they cared about their animals' welfare for emotional reasons but also for financial reasons. Their livelihood depends on their farm animals. Thus, concern for pets' safety creates a significant barrier for women, preventing them from seeking safe refuge from abuse (Ascione et al., 1997a; Faver & Strand, 2003b; Kogan et al., 2004).

Another reason to pay serious attention to animal abuse is that it may also be an indicator that the violence may be escalating and becoming more lethal. Ascione and his colleagues (1997a) discovered that the severity of physical abuse was associated with threats and actual harm to pets. In other words, those who threatened or actually harmed their pets more severely physically abused their partners than comparison women in the community. On the other hand, Walton-Moss and colleagues (2005) found no evidence that pet abuse was associated with lethality.

Witnessing cruelty to animals may desensitize children to violence against humans (Flynn, 2000c). Children exposed to pet abuse are likely to be traumatized. Seeing a loved family pet being harmed, especially by a parent, is disturbing. Children feel helpless to protect their pet and sometimes experience emotional detachment and a reduced capacity for empathy in order to psychologically cope with the trauma (Ascione, 1993). Exposure to both parent and pet abuse teaches some children that violence is acceptable (Ascione et al., 1997b). There is some evidence that suggests that children who witness cruelty to animals are more likely to engage in abusing animals themselves (Flynn, 1999). Almost one-third of households in DeViney et al.'s (1983) early work reported that children had been involved in terrorizing or harming the family pet. Addressing cruelty to animals within families may promote earlier identification of families in need of support or children in need of protection.

There may be long-term effects as well. Committing animal abuse as a child is associated with other forms of interpersonal aggression in adulthood. Flynn (1999) investigated early animal abuse and its consequences in a sample of 267 undergraduate students. He found that participants who had committed childhood acts of animal abuse were significantly more likely to support corporal punishment of children, and to approve of a husband slapping his wife as a means of control than participants who had never committed animal abuse in their childhoods even after controlling for age, gender, childhood experience with physical punishment, and biblical literalism. These factors may contribute to the intergenerational cycle of violence–children repeating the aggressive dynamics in their own adult lives.

Research has also shown that there is an association between childhood cruelty to animals and later criminal behavior. Arluke, Levin, Luke, and Ascione (1999) found that 70% of those who abused animals also committed at least one other criminal offense compared to only 22% of the control group. Although the evidence is largely anecdotal and based on case studies (the veracity is unquestioned by criminologists and individuals in law enforcement agencies) aggressive criminals more frequently committed acts of animal cruelty in their childhoods than non-aggressive criminals (Miller & Knutson, 1997; Ponder & Lockwood, 2000). Data collected retrospectively from men who were convicted felons (Miller & Knutson, 1997) and convicted serial killers show that the many of these individuals had been cruel to animals in their childhoods (Kellert & Felthous, 1985; Ressler, Burgess, & Douglas, 1988). Cruelty to animals is one of the symptoms of childhood conduct disorder included in the Diagnostic and Statistical Manual of Mental Disorders, 4th edition (DSM-IV; American Psychiatric Association, 1994). It is one symptom in a triad of symptoms (i.e., fire setting, enuresis, and cruelty to animals) that suggest serious psychopathology in children. There is some contrary evidence. Arluke and his colleagues (1999) found that although there were associations between animal cruelty and other forms of violence, early convictions of animal abuse were no more likely to be preceded or followed by convictions of violent interpersonal offences in men.

IMPLICATIONS FOR PROFESSIONALS WORKING WITH WOMEN, CHILDREN, FAMILIES AND ANIMALS

Acknowledging the Role of Pets in Women's and Children's Lives

Concern over pets is a significant barrier for women wanting to leave abusive homes. Women both delay seeking shelter because of their pets and worry about their pets when they do leave them behind. This worry and anxiety comes at a time when they are already dealing with considerable trauma and crises. Professionals who work with abused women need to understand the role of pets in families, and the emotional stress placed upon women leaving their beloved pets at home with the abuser. Educating professionals about the emotional stress experienced by women is critical to enhance the healing process (Ascione, 1998; Quinlisk, 1999). Given that many people consider their pets to be family members, shelter workers need to be respectful of women's concerns and worries over their pets that are often a strong source of emotional support.

Service providers need to offer battered women an opportunity to discuss their concerns about their pets. Research has shown that although the majority of shelter staff reported their clients talked about pet abuse, only a small percentage of shelters actually asked questions about pets during their intake interview (Ascione et al., 1997b). Shelter workers need to inquire whether women have pets, whether their pets have been threatened or harmed, and whether they are worried about leaving their pets with their partners. Questions of this nature need to be included on intake assessment forms. Asking questions allows women to express their worries and concerns in a safe and supportive environment and provides shelter staff the opportunity to assist women to make arrangements to ensure their pets' safety.

Risk assessment forms need to include questions about pet abuse. Professionals working within the context of family violence need to offer more attention to cruelty to animals since it may be an indicator that physical violence may be increasing. Protocols that include a brief question or two about animal abuse during intake interviews and crisis calls may help assess the partner's capacity for more serious physical violence and lethality. It is important for shelter workers to incorporate information about animal welfare in safety planning since there may be repeated visits to shelters and many crisis calls before women make the decision to leave abusive partners. Making arrangements for pets' safety needs to be included in safety planning for women attempting to leave abusive relationships to remove this barrier to leaving.

Creating Innovative Programs to Provide Safe Havens for Pets

Partnerships with local humane societies and the development and recruitment of temporary foster placement programs for pets may facilitate a woman's decision to leave an abusive home. In Canada, for example, several child welfare organizations have, or are working toward, partnerships with local humane societies as a form of *institutional cooperation* to maximize services for children, women, and animals (Zilney & Zilney, 2005). If the services are available, more women could potentially take advantage and leave their abusive homes. Offering women a safe place for their pets may help them in their decision-making when faced with abuse or at least eliminate this barrier for women.

An animal foster program has been initiated in one Colorado safehouse for abused women and their children (Kogan et al., 2004). The program has fostered more than 90 animals over a 4-year period. Animals remain in foster care in a separate location from the shelter for one week longer than the woman's stay. Women who accessed the foster program frequently reported that they would not have left their partners without somewhere to take their pets (Kogan et al., 2004).

Collaboration Among Different Service Delivery Professionals to Better Identify Violent Families

Collaborative approaches are needed between human and animal welfare organizations to better identify violent homes, particularly homes experiencing multiple forms of violence. Through greater collaboration between human and animal welfare organizations, stronger prevention efforts and service delivery for victims and survivors of family violence may occur (Faver & Strand, 2003b). Policies are needed to enable sharing of information between both groups of professionals to encourage a more effective response to human and animal victims of violence (Flynn, 2000c).

Cross-training and cross-referrals between animal control officers and human service professionals is an innovative approach that encourages collaboration in dealing with family violence and pet abuse (Flynn, 2000c). Cross-training programs promote information sharing and interactions among law enforcement, protective services, and animal welfare organizations. This helps to detect and prevent violence against children and animals (Boat, 1995). For example, child protection workers would observe the condition of pets while investigating child abuse cases and animal welfare workers would observe the well-being of children while investigating reported cases of animal abuse (Boat, 1995). In California, for example, animal control officers are mandated to report suspected child abuse cases encountered in the general performance of their duties (Arkow, 1996). In some states, veterinarians are considered health professionals and mandated to report suspected child abuse (Becker & French, 2004). Policies that foster information sharing among the human service and animal welfare professionals could result in a more effective response to all victims of violence (Flynn, 2000c).

Police officers need to inform both child protection services and humane societies when dealing with domestic violence cases where child abuse or animal abuse is suspected. Human service professionals in each social service organization need to be aware of all other forms of abuse toward different family members so that they can refer people to the appropriate organizations.

Health care providers have a vital role in recognizing and screening for family violence when providing routine exams or medical treatment. Abuse has serious consequences for physical, emotional, and social health and well being (Campbell, 2000; World Health Organization, 2002). In addition to the acute injuries such as fractures and lacerations, women often experience chronic health problems related to the abuse. Living with the tension, chronic stress, fear, and humiliation take an incredible toll on women's emotional health (Dobash & Dobash, 1992; Walker, 1979). In an effort to cope with the abuse, some women use alcohol or drugs, which only leads to further health and social problems. Abused children experience many of the same health problems as abused women (Gary & Humphreys, 2004). Children exposed to abuse in their family have similar problems to children who are themselves physically abused. They experience more social, emotional, and physical health problems than non-exposed children (Onyskiw, 2002; Onyskiw, 2003). Sometimes, these children are inadvertently injured during the abusive episodes as they try to protect the victim. Thus, abused women and children seek medical attention for health problems directly related to the abuse and secondary to the abuse. While some women neglect to seek care for themselves, almost all women will seek medical attention for their children. Often, the pediatric setting may be women's only point of access to health care (National Association of Children's Hospitals and Related Institutions, 2004; Siegel et al., 2003). It is important that health care providers in all acute and community settings be cognizant of the connections among all forms of abuse to better respond to violence in families.

Health care providers need to be particularly vigilant when people suffer animal-related injuries. Pets often react to being teased or terrorized by lashing out and harming humans. When comparing the rate of injuries in families that abused their pets to families that did not abuse their pets, DeViney and her colleagues (1983) found that 69% of homes with abused pets also had a family member who had been injured by the pet. The rate of injuries in non-pet-abusing homes was only 6%. Health care providers need to inquire about violence at home when people seek care for injuries from their own pets.

Knowledge on the link between family violence and animal abuse merits the attention of social workers in order to better recognize the different forms of violence that may exist in the same family (Faver & Strand, 2003). Other professionals such as teachers, child and adult protection workers, home care workers, and lawyers need to better understand the link between family violence and pet abuse in order to provide a more holistic, or *systems* approach to the issue of family violence (Faver & Strand, 2003). All practitioners may benefit from knowledge of the differing aspects and contributing factors to family violence (Tajima, 2004). When workers in one profession are able to identify indicators of family violence primarily treated by another professional, they are more likely to notify the other organization about possible abuse occurring in the home. A better understanding of the connections among all forms of violence would better inform our prevention efforts.

Multi-disciplinary community-based partnerships between health practitioners, social service workers, child protection workers, and law enforcement personnel are being implemented and evaluated (Kantor & Little, 2003; Onyskiw, Harrison, Spady, & McConnan, 1999). These collaborations have been reported to provide families with more immediate support during stressful times, improve batterer accountability, and improve linkages to community resources. The community-based approach makes access to services easier for clients, particularly for those individuals who were more socially isolated. Multidisciplinary, community-based models of service delivery may help better identify families characterized by multiple forms of violence and contribute to a more effective and compassionate response to these vulnerable families.

CONCLUSION

Although scientific studies of the connections between family violence and abuse of family pets are still relatively few in number, their strength lies in the fact that they come from a variety of data sources, were conducted by different investigators from different disciplines, and show remarkable consistency in their findings. Evidence gleaned from these studies suggests that cruelty to animals occurs disproportionately in violent families. Further, there is a link between the treatment of animals and the abuse of humans in vulnerable families. This link has important implications for many human and social service professionals who work with women, children, families and animals. There is sufficient evidence to warrant further investigation to better understand the nature of this serious problem and the human-animal connections and to change current policies and practices to provide a more comprehensive and coordinated approach to identifying and responding to individuals in vulnerable families.

AUTHOR NOTE

Judee E. Onyskiw, RN, PhD, is an educator and research advisor in the Faculty of Health and Community Studies at MacEwan College in Edmonton, Alberta. Prior to her current position, she was a Canada Research Chair in Family Violence and Health at the University of New Brunswick. Her research has primarily involved examining the impact of exposure to family violence on children's health, well-being, and social development and identifying factors that provide vulnerable children with some resilience.

The project was supported, in part, with a grant from the New Brunswick Innovation Foundation and the New Brunswick Department of Training and Employment while the author was a Canada Research Chair in Family Violence and Health at the University of New Brunswick.

The author would like to gratefully acknowledge Dianne Birt for her assistance on this project and Marilyn Merritt-Gray for her thoughtful review of this manuscript.

REFERENCES

Adams, C. J. (1998). Bringing peace home: A feminist philosophical perspective on the abuse of women, children and animals. In R. Lockwood & F. R. Ascione (Eds.), *Cruelty to animals and interpersonal violence: Readings in research and application* (pp. 318-340). West Lafayette, IN: Purdue University Press.

Agnew, R. (1998). The causes of animal abuse: A social-psychological analysis. *Theoretical Criminology, 2*(2), 177-209.

Albert, A., & Bulcroft, K. (1988). Pets, families, and the life course. *Journal of Marriage and the Family, 50,* 543-552.

American Psychiatric Association. (1994). *Diagnostic and statistical manual of mental disorders* (4th ed.). Washington, DC: Author.

American Veterinary Association. (1997). *U.S. pet ownership and demographic sourcebook.* Schaumburg, IL: Author.

Anaya, F. L. (2004). The relationship between child abuse and domestic violence in two groups of battered women. *Digital Dissertations, Section A: Humanities and Social Sciences, 64* (9-A), 3495.

Appel, A. E., & Holden, G. W. (1998). The co-occurrence of spouse and physical child abuse: A review and appraisal. *Journal of Family Psychology, 12*(4), 578-599.

Arkow, P. (1996). The relationship between animal abuse and other forms of family violence. *Family Violence and Sexual Assault Bulletin, 12,* 29-34.

Arluke, A., Levin, J., Luke, C., & Ascione, F. (1999). The relationship of animal abuse to violence and other forms of antisocial behavior. *Journal of Interpersonal Violence, 14*(9), 963-975.

Ascione, F. R. (1993). Children who are cruel to animals: A review of research and implications for developmental psychopathology. *Anthrozoos, 5*(4), 226-247.

Ascione, F. R. (1998). Battered women's reports of their partners' and their children's cruelty to animals. *Journal of Emotional Abuse, 1*(1), 119-133.

Ascione, F. R., Weber, C. V., & Wood, D. S. (1997a). *Animal welfare and domestic violence.* Final report submitted to the Geraldine R. Dodge Foundation.

Ascione, F. R., Weber, C. V., & Wood, D. S. (1997b). The abuse of animals and domestic violence: A national survey of shelters for women who are battered. *Society & Animals, 5*(3), 205-218.

Becker, F., & French, L. (2004). Making the links: Child abuse, animal cruelty and domestic violence. *Child Abuse Review, 13,* 399-414.

Beirne, P. (2002). Criminology and animal studies: A sociological view. *Society & Animals, 10*(4), 381-386.

Boat, B. W. (1995). The relationship between violence to children and violence to animals: An ignored link? *Journal of Interpersonal Violence, 10*(4), 229-235.

Bremner, R. H. (Ed.). (1970). *Children and youth in America: A documentary history.* (Vols. 1-2). Cambridge, MA: Harvard University Press.

Campbell, J. C. (2000). Promise and perils of surveillance in addressing violence against women. *Violence Against Women, 6*(7), 705-727.

Carlisle-Frank, P., Frank, J. M., & Nielsen, L. (2004). Selective battering of the family pet. *Anthrozoos, 17*(1), 26-42.

Carmack, B. J. (1985). The effects on family members and functioning after the death of a pet. *Marriage and Family Review, 8*(3/4), 149-161.

Child Abuse Prevention and Treatment Act, Public Law 93-247,42 U.S.C. § 5101 (1974).

Code, L. (1993). Feminist theory. In S. Burt, L. Code, & L. Dorney (Eds.), *Changing patterns: Women in Canada* (2nd ed., pp. 19-58). Toronto: McClelland & Steward.

Cole, S. G. (1993). Child battery. In B. J. Fox (Ed.), *Family patterns: Gender relations* (pp. 318-329). Toronto: Oxford University Press.

Counts, D. A., Brown, J. K., & Campbell, J. C. (Eds.). (1999). *To have and to hit: Cultural analysis of the beating of wives.* Bloomington, IL: University of Illinois.

Crook, A. (September, 2005). *Recognizing and addressing suspected animal abuse.* Proceeding at the Conference on Animal Abuse and Family Violence: Building a Community Response. Sir James Dunn Animal Welfare Centre, University of Prince Edward Island, Atlantic Veterinary College, Charlottetown, Prince Edward Island, Canada.

DeKeseredy, W. S. (2000). Current controversies on defining nonlethal violence against women in intimate heterosexual relationships. *Violence Against Women, 6*(7), 728-746.

DeViney, E., Dickert, J., & Lockwood, R. (1983). The care of pets within child abusing families. *International Journal of the Study of Animal Problems, 4*(4), 321-329.

Dobash, R. E., & Dobash, R. (1979). *Violence against wives: A case against the patriarchy.* New York: Free Press.

Dobash, R. E., & Dobash, R. (Eds.). (1992). *Rethinking violence against women.* London: Sage.

Doherty, D., & Hornosty, J. (2004). Abuse in a rural and farm context. In M. L. Sterling, C. A. Cameron, N. Nason-Clark, & B. Miedema (Eds.), *Understanding abuse: Partnering for change* (pp. 55-81). Toronto: University of Toronto Press.

Echlin, C., & Marshall, L. (1995). Child protection services for children of battered women. In E. Peled, P. G. Jaffe, & J. L. Edleson (Eds.), *Ending the cycle of violence: Community responses to children of battered women* (pp. 170-185). London: Sage.

Edleson, J. L. (1999). The overlap between child maltreatment and woman battering. *Violence Against Women, 5*(2), 134-154.

Faver, C. A., & Strand, E. B. (2003a). To leave or stay? Battered women's concern for vulnerable pets. *Journal of Interpersonal Violence, 18*(12), 1367-1377.

Faver, C. A., & Strand, E. B. (2003b). Domestic violence and animal cruelty: Untangling the web. *Journal of Social Work Education, 39*(2), 237-253.

Favre, D., & Tsang, V. (1993). The development of anti-cruelty laws during the 1800s. *Detroit College of Law Review, 1*, 1-35.

Flynn, C. P. (1999). Animal abuse in childhood and later support for interpersonal violence in families. *Society & Animals, 7*(2), 161-172.

Flynn, C. P. (2000a). Woman's best friend: Pet abuse and the role of companion animals in the lives of battered women. *Violence Against Women, 6*(2), 162-177.

Flynn, C. P. (2000b). Battered women and their animal companions: Symbolic interaction between human and nonhuman animals. *Society & Animals, 8*(2), 99-127.

Flynn, C. P. (2000c). Why family professionals can no longer ignore violence toward animals. *Family Relations, 49*(1), 87-95.

Folsom, W. S., Christensen, M. L., Avery, L., & Moore, C. (2003). The co-occurrence of child abuse and domestic violence: An issue of service delivery for social service professionals. *Child and Adolescent Social Work Journal, 20*(5), 375-387.

Gary, F., & Humphreys, J. (2004). Nursing care of abused children. In J. Campbell & J. Humphreys (Eds.), *Family violence and nursing practice* (pp. 252-287). New York: Lippincott, Williams, & Wilkins.

Gelles, R. J. (2000a). Estimating the incidence and prevalence of violence against women. *Violence Against Women, 6*(7), 784-804.

Gelles, R. J. (2000b). Public policy for violence against women: 30 years of successes and remaining challenges. *Journal of Preventive Medicine, 19*(4), 298-301.

Gordon, M. (2000). Definitional issues in violence against women: Surveillance research from a violence research perspective. *Violence Against Women, 6*(7), 747-783.

Hutton, J. S. (1983). Animal abuse a diagnostic approach in social work: A pilot study (reprinted). In R. Lockwood & F. R. Ascione (Eds.), *Cruelty to animals and interpersonal violence: Readings in research and application* (pp. 415-420). West Lafayette, IN: Purdue University Press.

Jacobson, N., & Gottman, J. (1998). *When men batter women: New insights into ending abusive relationships.* New York: Simon and Schuster.

Johnson, H. (1996). *Dangerous domains: Violence against women in Canada.* Toronto: Neilson Canada.

Jones, A. S., Gielen, A. C., Campbell, J. C., Schollenberger, J., Dienemann, J. A., Kub, J., et al. (1999). Annual and lifetime prevalence of partner abuse in a sample of female HMO enrollees. *Women's Health Issues, 9*(6), 295-305.

Kantor, G. K., & Little, L. (2003). Defining the boundaries of child neglect: When does domestic violence equate with parental failure to protect? *Journal of Interpersonal Violence, 18*(4), 338-355.

Kellert, S., & Felthous, A. R. (1985). Childhood cruelty towards animals among criminals and non criminals. In R. Lockwood & F. R. Ascione (Eds.), *Cruelty to animals and interpersonal violence: Readings in research and application* (pp. 194-210). West Lafayette, IN: Purdue University Press.

Kempe, C. H., Silverman, F. N., Steele, B., Droemueller, W., & Silver, H. K. (1962). The battered child syndrome. *Journal of the American Medical Association, 181*, 17-24.

Kogan, L. R., McConnell, S., Schoenfeld-Tacher, R., & Jansen-Lock, P. (2004). Crosstrails: A unique foster program to provide safety for pets of women in safehouses. *Violence Against Women, 10*(4), 418-434.

Lee, L. C., Kotch, J. B., & Cox, C. E. (2004). Child maltreatment in families experiencing domestic violence. *Violence and Victims, 19*(5), 573-591.

Lewandowski, L. A., McFarlane, J., Campbell, J. C., Gary, F., & Barenski, C. (2004). "He killed my mommy!" Murder or attempted murder of a child's mother. *Journal of Family Violence, 19*(4), 211-220.

McIntosh, S. C. (2001). Exploring the links between animal abuse and family violence. *The Latham Letter, XXII*, 14-16.

McKay, M. M. (1994). The link between domestic violence and child abuse: Assessment and treatment considerations. *Child Welfare, 73*(1), 29-39.

Miller, K. S., & Knutson, J. F. (1997). Reports of severe physical punishment and exposure to animal cruelty by inmates convicted of felonies and by university students. *Child Abuse & Neglect, 21*(1), 59-82.

National Association of Children's Hospitals and Related Institutions (2004). Understanding the link between child abuse and domestic violence: An essential part of family-centered care. *NACHRI Profile Series,* May 4-15.

Onyskiw, J. E. (2002). Health and the use of health services of children exposed to violence in their families. *Canadian Journal of Public Health, 93*(6), 416-420.

Onyskiw, J. E. (2003). Domestic violence and children's adjustment: A review of research. *Journal of Emotional Abuse, 3*(1/2), 11-45.

Onyskiw, J. E. (2005). A concept analysis of abuse. In J. R. Cutcliffe & H. McKenna (Eds.), *The essential concepts of nursing* (pp. 15-31). London: Elsevier.

Onyskiw, J. E., Harrison, M., Spady, D., & McConnan, L. (1999). Formative evaluation of a collaborative community-based child abuse prevention project. *Child Abuse and Neglect, 23*(11), 1069-1081.

Osofsky, J. D. (2003). Prevalence of children's exposure to domestic violence and child maltreatment: Implications for prevention and intervention. *Clinical Child and Family Psychology Review, 6*(3), 161-170.

Ponder, C., & Lockwood, R. (2000). Programs educate law enforcement on link between animal cruelty and domestic violence. *The Police Chief, LXVII*(11), 31-36.

Quinlisk, J. A. (1999). Animal abuse and family violence. In F. R. Ascione & P. Arkow (Eds.), *Child abuse, domestic violence, and animal abuse: Linking the circles of compassion for prevention an intervention* (pp. 168-175). West Layette, IN: Purdue University Press.

Renzelli C. M. (1992). *Violent betrayal: Partner abuse in lesbian relationships.* Newbury Park, CA: Sage.

Ressler, R. K., Burgess, A. W., & Douglas, J. E. (1988). *Sexual homicide: Patterns and motives.* Lexington, MA: Lexington Books.

Ross, S. M. (1996). Risk of physical abuse to children of spouse abusing parents. *Child Abuse and Neglect, 20,* 589-598.

Saltzmann, L. E., Fanslow, J. L., McMahon, P. M., & Shelley, G. A. (1999). *Intimate partner violence surveillance: Uniform definitions and recommended data elements, Version 1.0.* Atlanta, GA: National Center for Injury Prevention and Control, Centers for Disease Prevention.

Siegel, R. M., Joseph, E. C., Routh, S. A., Mendel, S. G., Jones, E., Ramesh, R. B., et al. (2003). Screening for domestic violence in the pediatric office: A multipractice experience. *Clinical Pediatrics, 42*(7), 599-602.

Solot, D. (1997). Untangling the animal abuse web. *Society & Animals, 5,* 257-265.

Stark, E., & Flitcraft, A. (1996). *Woman at risk: Domestic violence and women's health.* Thousand Oaks, CA: Sage.

Statistics Canada. (2005). *Family violence in Canada: A statistical profile* (Canadian Centre for Justice Statistics Publication No. 85-224-XIE). Ottawa, Ontario: Author.

Suthers-McCabe, M. (2005, September). *Role of veterinarians in reporting child and animal abuse.* Proceeding at the Conference on Animal Abuse and Family Violence: Building a Community Response. Sir James Dunn Animal Welfare Centre,

University of Prince Edward Island, Atlantic Veterinary College, Charlottetown, Prince Edward Island, Canada.

Tajima, E. A. (2000). The relative importance of wife abuse as a risk factor for violence against children. *Child Abuse and Neglect, 24*(11), 1383-1398.

Tajima, E. A. (2004). Correlates of the co-occurrence of wife abuse and child abuse among a representative sample. *Journal of Family Violence, 19*(6), 399-410.

Tjaden, P., & Thoennes, N. (2000). *Extent, nature, and consequences of intimate partner violence: Findings from the National Violence Against Women Survey.* Washington, DC: U.S. Department of Justice.

United States Department of Justice. (2005). *Family violence statistics: Including statistics on strangers and acquaintances.* (Office of Justice Programs Publication No. 207846). Washington, DC: Author.

Walker, L. E. (1979). *The battered woman.* New York: Harper & Row.

Walton-Moss, B. J., Manganello, J., Frye, V., & Campbell, J. C. (2005). Risk factors for intimate partner violence and associated injury among urban women. *Journal of Community Health, 30*(5), 377-389.

World Health Organization. (2002). *World report on violence and health.* Geneva: Author.

Yllo, K. A. (1993). Through a feminist lens: Gender, power, and violence. In R. J. Gelles & D. R. Loseke (Eds.), *Current controversies on family violence* (pp. 47-62). London: Sage.

Zilney, L. A., & Zilney, M. (2005). Reunification of child and animal welfare agencies: Cross-reporting of abuse in Wellington County, Ontario. *Child Welfare, 84*(1), 47-66.

Zink, T., Kamine, D., Musk, L., Sill, M., Field, V., & Putman, F. (2004). What are providers' reporting requirements for children who witness domestic violence? *Clinical Pediatrics, 43*(5), 449-460.

doi:10.1300/J135v07n03_02

Cruelty to Animals
and the Short- and Long-Term Impact
on Victims

Karen D. Schaefer

SUMMARY. Research indicates that various types of childhood abuse occurring in violent families (e.g., physical or emotional abuse) do not happen in isolation. Clients often describe experiencing multiple forms of maltreatment in childhood, and research indicates an increased severity of symptoms with each added form of abuse. Regardless of the kinds of abuse perpetrated against them, clients report similar short- and long-term effects. It is proposed that witnessing, being threatened with, or forced to commit animal abuse constitutes an important form of abuse. Similar to the impact of other forms of abuse, comparable short- and long-term effects could exist for both the human and nonhuman survivors of animal abuse. Recommendations for addressing the trauma of animal abuse are offered. doi:10.1300/J135v07n03_03 *[Article copies available for a fee from The Haworth Document Delivery Service: 1-800-HAWORTH. E-mail address: <docdelivery@haworthpress.com> Website: <http://www.HaworthPress.com>* © *2007 by The Haworth Press. All rights reserved.]*

Address correspondence to: Karen D. Schaefer, PhD, Counseling Center, Garcia Annex, MSC 3575, New Mexico State University, Las Cruces, NM 88003 (E-mail: kschaefe@nmsu.edu).

[Haworth co-indexing entry note]: "Cruelty to Animals and the Short- and Long-Term Impact on Victims." Schaefer, Karen D. Co-published simultaneously in *Journal of Emotional Abuse* (The Haworth Maltreatment & Trauma Press, an imprint of The Haworth Press) Vol. 7, No. 3, 2007, pp. 31-57; and: *Animal Abuse and Family Violence: Linkages, Research, and Implications for Professional Practice* (ed: Marti T. Loring, Robert Geffner, and Janessa Marsh) The Haworth Maltreatment & Trauma Press, an imprint of The Haworth Press, 2007, pp. 31-57. Single or multiple copies of this article are available for a fee from The Haworth Document Delivery Service [1-800-HAWORTH, 9:00 a.m. - 5:00 p.m. (EST). E-mail address: docdelivery@haworthpress.com].

KEYWORDS. Animal abuse, trauma, short- and long-term effects

It is now recognized in the professional literature that abuse does not occur in a singular manner. The various forms of abuse, physical, sexual, emotional, and neglect, might happen simultaneously, rather than take place as separate and distinct occurrences. Thus, researchers recognize that it is unusual for victims to experience only one form of abuse or neglect. Quite often, multiple forms of maltreatment are occurring within the same family. For example, a child who witnesses domestic violence might also experience physical and emotional abuse concurrently (Arata, Langhinrichsen-Rohling, Bowers, & O'Farrill-Swails, 2005; Cox, Kotch, & Everson, 2003; Johnson et al., 2002).

The impact of living in an abusive family environment has potential short- and long-term effects for the child, adolescent, and adult victim. A number of studies are indicating that there is an additive effect such that the more forms of abuse and neglect occurring within a family, the greater the associated distress and traumatic symptoms the victim might experience (Cox et al., 2003; Dong, Anda, Dube, Giles, & Felitti, 2003; Edwards, Holden, Felitti, & Anda, 2003; McGuigan & Middlemiss, 2005; Runyon & Kenny, 2002; Ystgaard, Hestetun, Loeb, & Mehlum, 2004).

One type of abuse that could occur in a violent family but is not often mentioned in the theoretical models or research literature pertaining to trauma is that of animal abuse. In this article, it is proposed that witnessing, being threatened with or forced to commit animal abuse is an additional form of maltreatment that could provoke short- and long-term effects for the victim. In a home environment where abuse is occurring, animal abuse is very likely to be a part of the family violence. A child witnessing the abuse of a beloved companion animal could be equally devastated as if they had experienced physical, sexual, emotional abuse or neglect. In fact, it is argued that animal abuse could actually constitute a form of physical, sexual, or emotional abuse. Finally, it is suggested that animal abuse taking place in a violent family where other forms of maltreatment are also taking place could add to the severity of a client's symptomology and psychological distress.

Therapists can draw upon existing theoretical frameworks and research pertinent to trauma victims to understand the effects animal abuse may have on an individual client. Case examples will be utilized to highlight theoretical concepts and research findings pertaining to the short- and long-term effects of abuse. It will be suggested that all of the various forms of direct or indirect (witnessing) abuse share similar effects on victims. Potential parallels between the effects of witnessing, being threatened with or forced to commit animal abuse and the multiple forms of abuse and neglect will be identified–not only for the human victims but also for the animal victims. Based upon what a healthy relationship between human and nonhuman animals might offer, treatment recommendations for assisting victims through the healing process will be proposed.

THEORETICAL BASIS FOR UNDERSTANDING THE EFFECTS OF ABUSE

Various models have been proposed to assist therapists in helping clients who have experienced the trauma associated with a number of different forms of abuse and neglect. For the purposes of this article, the psychological trauma model of Herman (1992) will be utilized to understand the impact of childhood abuse. Herman proposes that trauma could be defined in a variety of ways and occurs in a number of settings (e.g., rape, marital battery, childhood abuse, prisoners of war, and concentration camp survivors). These harmful experiences share the common feature that all involve the experience of terror, violence, and abuse. This model calls attention to the fact that witnesses as well as direct victims can experience the effects of trauma. The notion that witnessing traumatic events can be victimizing in itself is supported in the work of several authors (e.g., Becker-Blease & Freyd, 2005; Graham-Bermann & Hughes, 1998; Kerig, Fedorowicz, Brown & Warren, 2000; Turner, Finkelhor & Ormrod, 2006).

Children who are faced with repeated incidents of abuse find ways of psychologically protecting themselves. These coping strategies allow the child to survive the trauma of abuse and associated experiences of helplessness, powerlessness, and lack of safety. Herman suggests that surviving abuse calls for learning and using skills that are fraught with the potential for healthy outcomes as well as unhealthy outcomes. For example, a survivor of sexual abuse might deal with the abuse by altering his or her mind and entering into a trance-like state, which would serve as a protective function at the time the abuse is occurring. If carried into adulthood, this strategy could pose problems later on in a victim's life.

When seeking therapy, survivors can present with an array of concerns: depression, heightened levels of anxiety, hypervigilance, suicidal thoughts or gestures, self-mutilation, feelings of shame, guilt, and blame, and interpersonal concerns (Herman, 1992). Given that therapists are often faced with helping abuse survivors who are presenting with a range and multitude of symptomotology, Herman suggests that the post-traumatic stress disorder (PTSD) diagnosis as described in the current DSM-IV diagnostic classification system (American Psychiatric Association, 2000) is too limited in capturing the experience of the person who is subjected to inescapable, prolonged and repeated trauma or abuse. She recommends that the numerous and varied psychological and physiological responses victims have to the trauma of abuse could be better understood by drawing upon a spectrum of post-traumatic disorders. This spectrum could range from a brief stress reaction, to the current conceptualization of PTSD, to what she describes as the "complex post-traumatic stress disorder" condition. The proposed complex post-traumatic stress disorder would be used to understand the symptomology of those clients who were exposed to inescapable, repeated and prolonged (months to years) periods of trauma and abuse.

The criteria for the complex post-traumatic stress disorder is based upon a categorization of the multiple symptoms that might occur as a survivor attempts to cope with chronic abuse. These symptoms are categorized as reflecting alterations in various aspects of the survivor's functioning and belief system. For example, the criteria of "alterations in consciousness" (p. 121) would account for the dissociative episodes an adult survivor of childhood sexual abuse might experience. Alterations in consciousness could also capture the reliving of past trauma by repeatedly experiencing intrusive recollections of the abuse. Other criteria that are proposed within the complex post-traumatic stress disorder would include alterations in: affect regulation (e.g., persistent dysphoria); self-perception (e.g., sense of helplessness, self-blame, defilement or stigma, different from others); the perception of the perpetrator (e.g., preoccupation with the relationship with the perpetrator); relations with others (e.g., isolation, withdrawal, struggle with intimacy); and systems of meaning (e.g., sense of hopelessness or despair).

Case Example #1

Alicia was a middle-aged, Caucasian client whose presenting concern for counseling was her desire to deal with the stress of being a single parent. She also wanted to learn how to be a more effective parent to her three children. Alicia was dealing with multiple roles and demands in her life, including being a student, employee, and mother. Alicia disclosed that she was an animal lover and believed that her children should have the experience of growing up with animals. In the course of counseling, Alicia described having a traumatic childhood–abandoned by her mother when she was one year old, she was raised by her father who was physically abusive. Alicia described how she used to cope with the abuse and neglect by retreating into fantasy and creating a safe and magical "world" where she was able to escape from the emotional and physical pain she was experiencing. Additionally, Alicia noted that her father tended to be neglectful of her needs as a child, leaving her up to her own devices to care for herself. Alicia could recall seeing the family dogs being neglected as well, to the point that several dogs died due to malnourishment.

Several months into the counseling, Alicia disclosed to her therapist that she had abused one of her cats because he had scratched her with his claws. She described feeling unreal and as though she was "not herself" as she put the cat into the freezer for a period of time and then threw him outside into a bucket full of water. When she eventually "came to" and recognized the cat's distress, she was appalled at what she had done to him. In discussing this with her counselor, it was discovered that Alicia had been collecting and hoarding animals. She had 20 animals of various species in her home even though she did not have the financial means to take care of them. Alicia expressed her strong fear that if she did not have the animals around to alternatively receive affection from and to serve as buffers for her frustration and anger, her children would become the next targets of her rage.

In this case example, Alicia described an episode of personalization when she was abusing her cat. The unreal feeling and sense that she was somehow detached from herself ("not herself") were familiar to her in that this is how she survived the abuse she experienced as a child. These coping strategies, which helped her to deal with the abuse and neglect, would be representations of the alterations in consciousness criteria of the complex post-traumatic stress disorder. As a child, Alicia used to escape to another world, and this ability was now negatively impacting her in a multitude of ways, including her awareness of when she was being abusive to another being.

Case Example #2

Chuck was a young Latino who was seeking therapy due to a growing awareness that his history of childhood sexual abuse was impacting the relationship with his girlfriend. He would have the need to occasionally isolate himself and withdraw from intimacy with his girlfriend but was unable to understand or find an explanation for this need. Chuck was also disturbed by his tendency to alternate between being explosively angry and inhibiting his anger. Chuck described coming from a home where his parents modeled very traditional gender role behaviors. His mother was a homemaker and his father was a rancher and an elder of the fundamental church of which the family were members.

Between the ages of 5 and 11, Chuck was repeatedly sexually abused by his father who also abused his two younger brothers. Chuck vividly recalled how his father threatened to kill his dog and younger brothers if he disclosed the abuse to anyone. On occasion, his father would punish Chuck's dog for some misbehavior Chuck had committed. Chuck often witnessed seeing his father hit and kick the dog and could still recall hearing the dog's cries. Chuck coped with the sexual abuse and the animal abuse he experienced by blaming himself and could experience powerful self-loathing, particularly when he was enraged with his father.

While in therapy, Chuck recounted an event that occurred when he was visiting his parents over the Labor Day holiday. Chuck's dog had attacked and killed his father's dog. Chuck was pleased that this occurred and that his father had to experience emotional suffering due to the loss. It was difficult for Chuck to allow himself to have empathy for the suffering his father's dog experienced prior to his death. At the time he reported this incident in a therapy session, he was unaware of how his pleasure over his father's pain might be related to the hurt and anger he felt that was associated with the past childhood abuse.

Drawing upon this case example, one can see how Chuck's shifting between explosive anger and inhibiting anger would be explained by the alterations in affect regulation criteria. It is noteworthy that when Chuck was abused as a child, he blamed himself, particularly when he experienced anger and rage toward his father. This self-blame is one way a child could understand why the abuse was occurring to him and is reflective of the alteration in self-perception that occurs in response to such trauma. Additionally, his tendency to isolate himself and withdraw from the relationship with his girlfriend would be indicative of alterations in his relations with others. Herman's model can provide the framework for conceptualizing the various short- and long-term effects therapists may hear from clients who report histories of childhood abuse. The model could also provide the bridge between the impact of the various forms of childhood abuse and the hypothesized impact of witnessing, being threatened with or forced to commit animal abuse as a child or adolescent.

SIMILARITY OF EFFECTS ACROSS ABUSE TYPES

Post-Traumatic Stress Symptoms

While there has been little research on the short- and long-term effects of witnessing, being threatened with or forced to commit animal abuse, much more research has been conducted on the short- and long-term effects of sexual, emotional, physical abuse and neglect. In support of Herman's model, many of the symptoms associated with post-traumatic stress disorder have been identified in studies that have been conducted on victims of sexual, physical, emotional abuse and neglect. Signs of post-traumatic stress disorder, such as experiencing flashbacks of the abuse, repetitive and intrusive thoughts and recollections, nightmares, and associated arousal symptoms, have been described by Briere and Elliott (1994) in their study of adult survivors of childhood sexual abuse. These same authors note that many of the survivors avoided triggers of the past abuse via emotional numbing, dissociation, derealization and depersonalization. Children and adolescent victims of physical abuse, neglect, or sexual abuse have been found to experience psychological symptoms associated with increased arousal such as hypervigilance, sleep disturbance, anxiety, or difficulty with concentration (Conte & Schuerman, 1987; Famularo, Kinscherff, & Fenton, 1992; Kerig et al., 2000).

Spertus, Yehuda, Wong, Halligan and Seremetis (2003) examined the impact of childhood emotional abuse and neglect on various indicators of psychological distress and physical symptomology experienced in adulthood. While controlling for physical abuse, sexual abuse, and other forms of childhood trauma, the authors found that emotional abuse and neglect were significant predictors for greater utilization of healthcare facilities (measured by number of visits to the doctor) and increased psychological distress as indicated by heightened levels of anxiety, somatization, depression, and post-traumatic stress disorder symptoms.

Experiencing abuse directly is only one form of trauma that a child might experience relative to family violence, and in the past 25 years, research has been conducted on the impact witnessing domestic violence has on children (Cunningham & Baker, 2004; Dutton, 2000). Graham-Bermann and Hughes (1998) state that studies of children who witness domestic violence indicate that 40-60% are at a higher risk for developing psychological problems when compared with children from nonviolent homes. A number of authors have noted that many child witnesses of domestic violence experience post-traumatic stress symptoms and could conceivably be diagnosed with the adult version of PTSD (Cunningham & Baker, 2004; Graham-Bermann & Levendosky, 1998; Kilpatrick, Litt, & Williams, 1997).

Given the nature of domestic violence, one can easily see how children could be so seriously impacted by being a witness that they might experience post-traumatic stress symptoms. In defining domestic violence, the child witness could see the abused parent experiencing ". . . harassment, emotional and psychological abuse, threats, violation of court orders (e.g., orders of protection, and no-contact orders), assault/battery, sex offenses, stalking, burglary, theft, embezzlement, destruction of property, kidnapping, child abduction, child abuse and homicide" (Turkel & Shaw, 2003, p. 1).

In their thorough review of the literature, Cunningham and Baker (2004) describe the potential impact witnessing domestic violence could have on children of differing developmental levels. These authors suggest that children of different age groups–infants/toddlers, preschoolers, school age and adolescents–will have differing abilities for coping with witnessing abuse as well as differing means of processing the experience and expressing their distress. For example, infants and toddlers have limited cognitive abilities for understanding what they might be experiencing when domestic violence is occurring. They also have limited abilities to express their distress (e.g., being "fussy," not eating or sleeping) when compared to older children who can express themselves verbally and have greater behavioral repertoires to convey their distress (i.e., post-traumatic play).

Difficulties with Intimacy

Given that abuse occurs within the context of a relationship, it makes a great deal of sense that a survivor of abuse would struggle with interpersonal relationships, particularly in questioning whether or not a relationship is going to provide emotional safety, security, and an opportunity to trust. Davis and Petretic-Jackson (2000) addressed how the long-term effects of child sexual abuse might impact adult relationships, including the development of intimacy and sexual functioning. Bricre and Elliott (1994) also comment on how abuse-related interpersonal difficulties may be exhibited later in life. Adult survivors of sexual abuse might struggle with distrust in others and experience ambivalence and fear related to the vulnerability necessary for developing intimacy in a relationship.

A qualitative study of the long-term impact of maternal emotional abuse indicated interpersonal problems that are similar to the research identifying the impact of physical abuse and neglect and sexual abuse (DeRobertis, 2004). Those who experienced maternal emotional abuse and neglect tended to engage in avoidant behaviors in relationships. Similar to the report of many sexual abuse survivors, these avoidant behaviors included having difficulty with trust and the internal struggle of wanting but being fearful of interpersonal intimacy. The subjects also reported experiencing a need to dominate and be in control in their relationships with others.

Internalizing Symptoms

In a parallel but slightly different approach from Herman's conceptualization of the array of symptoms survivors might present with, some research on physically abused and neglected or sexually abused children has focused on "internalizing symptoms" such as depression, anxiety, suicidality, PTSD symptoms, self-destructive behaviors, and self-blame. A number of studies have reported that victims of childhood sexual abuse and physical abuse and neglect might experience increased susceptibility to behaviors such as drug and alcohol abuse, bulimia, suicidal ideation and attempts, self-mutilation, and engaging in risky behaviors (Briere & Elliott, 1994; Dube et al., 2005; Kendler, Bulik, Silberg, Hettema, Myers, & Prescott, 2000; Lansford, Dodge, Pettit, Bates, Crozier, & Kaplow, 2002; Swanston, Plunkett, O'Toole, Shrimpton, Parkinson, & Oates, 2003; Tyler, 2002; Ystgaard et al., 2004). In DeRobertis' (2004) study of emotional abuse, a number of the victims were engaging in "internalizing behaviors," which was indicated by depression and a tendency to engage in self-destructive behaviors as a means of expressing anger and serving as a cry for help. The subjects in DeRobertis' sample experienced low self-worth, inadequacy, and a powerful sense of shame associated with the abuse.

It is not surprising that research supports the notion that the internalizing symptoms associated with abuse and neglect can last years. In their 12-year longitudinal study of the long-term effects of physical abuse, Lansford et al. (2002) discovered that adolescents who had been abused prior to age five had numerous academic difficulties, including lower grades and standardized test scores. The adolescents were also absent and suspended from school much more frequently than the nonabused control group. In a number of studies, these long-term effects have been found to lead to negative mental health outcomes, including major depression, generalized anxiety, conduct disorder or panic disorder (Dinwiddie et al., 2000; Kendler et al., 2000; Spataro, Mullen, Burgess, Wells, & Moss, 2004; Windom, DuMont, & Czaja, 2007). In addressing adjustment in adulthood, Steel, Sanna, Hammond, Whipple, and Cross (2004) note that poorer adjustment occurs in those survivors who "internalize" the abuse, such that they attribute the blame of the abuse to themselves.

Externalizing Symptoms

Studies have also focused on "externalizing symptoms" such as antisocial behaviors, aggression, hostility, and disruptive social relationships (see for example, Valle & Silovsky, 2002). Conceptualizing symptoms as being either "internalizing" or "externalizing" can easily be adapted to the criteria described by Herman as it pertains to a diagnosis of complex post-traumatic disorder. Clearly, the internalizing symptom of depression could be considered an alteration in affect regulation, whereas the externalizing symptom of disruptive social relationships could be considered an alteration in relations with others.

Graham-Bermann and Hughes (1998) summarized research that indicated that children of battered women exhibit both internalizing and externalizing behavior problems. Indeed, McFarlane, Groff, O'Brien and Watson (2003) found that children in their sample who had been exposed to domestic violence exhibited higher levels of internalizing, externalizing, and total behavior problem when compared to "not exposed" peers who had not witnessed domestic violence. This finding held true regardless of the age, race, or ethnicity of the child. Gender appears to be an important factor to consider when assessing the effects of witnessing domestic violence. Edleson (1999) noted that much of the research indicates that boys who witness domestic violence are more inclined to experience externalizing behavioral problems when compared to girls who express more internalized problems.

Most importantly for the purposes of this article, Baldry (2003) assessed the effects of both witnessing domestic violence as well as witnessing animal abuse committed by a parent on externalizing problems as exhibited by adolescents who had committed animal abuse. In this study, Baldry gathered data from 1,396 adolescents and found that 47%

reported that their parents had been violent with one another at least once. Both mothers and fathers were offenders of the domestic violence. Of the youth that acknowledged having committed some form of abuse with an animal (1/2 of the sample), almost all reported higher levels of exposure to both domestic violence and witnessing animal abuse committed by their parents. Male adolescent subjects were six times more likely to commit animal abuse themselves if their mother had also committed animal abuse. This study did not examine the internalizing problems that could occur with youth who witnessed domestic violence and/or animal abuse committed by their parents.

It is important to note that many of the studies addressing short- and long-term effects attempted to examine each form of abuse–physical abuse or neglect and sexual abuse–independently of one another. It has been proposed that this separation might be a false one such that where one form of abuse exists within a family, so might other forms of abuse. For example, emotional abuse and neglect have been examined relative to their impact on victims, and while it can occur independently of physical abuse and neglect and sexual abuse, Garbarino, Guttman and Seeley (1986) suggest that emotional abuse and neglect underlies all of the various forms of abuse and neglect. With this in mind, researchers are beginning to examine the impact many forms of abuse may have on victims.

Impact of Multiple Forms of Maltreatment

It appears that abuse does not occur on a singular level–where there is one form of abuse and neglect, there are often multiple forms of abuse and neglect. Ney, Fung and Wickett (1994) examined the impact of differing types of abuse and neglect and found that in less than 5% of their subjects, the abuse occurred by itself. Additionally, a number of studies have clearly indicated that there is an additive effect, such that the more forms of abuse and neglect one experiences, the more severe the symptomotology and psychological distress (Cox et al., 2003; Dong et al., 2003; Edwards et al., 2003; Turner et al., 2006). These authors have found that multiple-abuse survivors have higher levels of depression (McGuigan & Middlemiss, 2005), suicidality (Arata et al., 2005), self-mutilation (Ystgaard et al., 2004), poor self-esteem, anxiety, aggression (Johnson et al., 2002), and post-traumatic stress symptoms (Runyon & Kenny, 2002).

The various forms of abuse examined in these studies included physical, sexual, and emotional abuse and neglect and witnessing domestic violence. Turner et al. (2006) explored the impact of multiple forms of trauma, stress, and adversity on mental health in their examination of child maltreatment. Abuse and neglect and witnessing domestic violence were considered to be victimizing traumas whereas serious illnesses, accidents, parental imprisonment, natural disasters, family members' substance abuse, parental arguing, and chronic teasing were considered to be non-victimizing traumas. These authors suggest that it is important that multiple, not single types of victimization or trauma, be examined in order to accurately attribute the specific short- or long-term effects that a victim might experience. It is noteworthy that none of these studies examined the impact of witnessing, being threatened with or forced to commit animal abuse as one of the forms of child maltreatment. Animal abuse could be a part of the additive and cumulative stress of being in a violent and chaotic family environment and could, therefore, intensify any symptoms a victim could experience.

In summary, it appears that survivors of abuse, whether witnesses or direct recipients of the abuse, are impacted in similar ways. One can see parallels in both the short- and long-term effects regardless of the type of abuse, including post-traumatic stress symptoms; interpersonal concerns; and internalizing symptoms as indicated by depression, anxiety, low self-esteem, self-blame, self-destructive, risk-taking or externalizing symptoms as indicated by behaviors such as inappropriate expression of anger or delinquency. This array of symptoms are often presenting concerns of clients with histories of abuse that a therapist needs to contend with and are certainly reflective of the complex post-traumatic syndrome described by Herman (1992).

THE IMPACT OF ANIMAL ABUSE

Animal Abuse as a Form of Physical, Sexual, or Emotional Abuse

One can easily find examples of how animal abuse itself could constitute forms of emotional, physical, sexual abuse and neglect. The American Humane Association includes terrorizing in its definition of emotional abuse and also mentions how pets can be used to terrorize a child: "Terrorizing can include placing the child or the child's loved one (such as a sibling, pet, or toy) in a dangerous or chaotic situation, or placing rigid or unrealistic expectations on the child with threats of harm if they are not met" (American Humane Association, 2006). Thus, living with the fear that one might lose their life as exemplified by see-ing their pet killed represents emotional abuse. Additionally, using the threat of abuse of a beloved animal to obtain cooperation or silence would be considered emotional abuse as well.

Animal abuse can constitute sexual abuse in the example where the victim is forced to participate in bestiality (Ascione, 2005). The sexu-ally abusive act of forcing a child, adolescent, or adult victim to perform bestiality could also be used to humiliate the victim and to ensure their silence. The use of animal abuse as a form of physical abuse of a child or adolescent victim is represented in the concept of "joint-discipline" (Raupp, Barlow & Oliver, 1997). This occurs when a pet is disciplined or punished for a child's behavior as well as the reverse–the child being punished via physical abuse for perceived misbehavior of the pet. An example of joint discipline would be the client who reported watching his father stand on the family puppy as a way of punishing the animal for the client's perceived "misbehavior" of not doing the assigned household chore he had been given to do. Given that animal abuse can be a form of emotional, sexual, and physical abuse, it would follow that victims would experience similar short- and long-term effects.

Potential Short- and Long-Term Effects of Animal Abuse

There are a few authors who directly mention the impact witnessing, being threatened with or forced to commit animal abuse might have on the intended victims. Research conducted by Arluke (2000) is one of the few studies that directly examined the secondary victimization that could be experienced by those whose companion animals were abused by either a family member or individual external to the family. Based upon semi-structured interviews of 18 adult females who reported intra- or extrafamilial abuse of a companion animal, Arluke compared their reactions to those who have been targets of other types of crimes. These women reported experiencing an acute crisis stage that included shock, disbelief, and rage upon learning about the abuse of the animal. After the initial shock, victims often reported experiencing complicated grief reactions and/or guilt, especially when their companion animal had been killed by the abuser. It is noteworthy that as victims attempted to learn to experience life without their companion animal, they experi-enced similar reactions of vulnerability as have been reported by vic-tims of other types of crimes. These women stated that they worried for months about retaliation from the offender for having reported the abuse and became vigilant about further abuse to their children as well as to their current companion animals. Finally, as the women coped with the abuse over a longer period of time, they attempted to find something positive of the experience. For example, several of the women were grateful that the abuse of their animal was the cause of their decision to finally leave an abusive marriage. Additionally, some reported experiencing stronger attachments to their companion animals because the animal had tried to protect them from abuse by their partner. While this study did not examine the short- or long-term impact that witnessing, being threatened with or forced to commit animal abuse could have if it occurred in childhood, it is a first effort to draw attention to the fact that animal abuse is a traumatic event that could cause similar reactions as those who were victims of other types of crimes.

Randour, Krinsk, and Wolf (2002) recommend that therapists need to assess for PTSD in children who witness animal cruelty. In the first case example mentioned in this article, the childhood neglect that caused Alicia's dogs to die from malnutrition was a vivid example to her of what might happen if she were unable to find the means to survive. One of the ways she coped with this threat to her survival was to escape to an imaginary world, which was indicative of the dissociative behavior seen with clients suffering from PTSD.

In her description of the traumatic effects of child abuse, Herman (1992) notes that threats of harm, injury, or death could be directed to a child's companion animal in an effort to solicit cooperation and silence the victim from disclosing the abuse to others. Consequently, she encourages therapists to attend to client's stories of animal abuse that occur within the family environment. Given that many trauma survivors describe the fear that their lives were in danger and the fear of dying, it is not a far cry to consider how seeing one's beloved pet being sadistically abused and/or killed would elicit the same fears. Witnessing, being threatened with or forced to commit animal abuse could be a part of the inescapable, repeated, and prolonged periods of trauma and abuse that underlie Herman's (1992) complex post-traumatic stress disorder syndrome. Consequently, one would expect to see similar coping strategies and the subsequent alterations in affect regulation (e.g., persistent dysphoria), consciousness (dissociation, reliving past trauma and experiencing intrusive memories), self-perception (sense of helplessness, self-blame, defilement or stigma, feeling different from others), perception of the perpetrator, relations with others (e.g., isolation, withdrawal, difficulty with trust) and in systems of meaning (hopelessness, despair) in the victims of animal abuse.

Ascione (1998, 2005) and Ascione, Friedrich, Heath, and Hayashi (2003) have proposed that experiencing abuse could increase a child or adolescent's risk of committing animal cruelty. Children and adolescents with histories of abuse and neglect and who are committing animal cruelty are exhibiting aggression, which is considered to be a form of externalizing behavior. There are several studies that did examine whether or not a subject had committed animal cruelty as a child and had witnessed it being done by another family member (Baldry, 2003; Baker, Boat, Grinvalsky & Geracioti, 1998; Flynn, 1999; Miller & Knutson, 1997). In these studies, the range of subjects who reported committing animal cruelty was from 10% to 51%; the range of subjects who reported witnessing animal cruelty was from 27% to 49%. In many of these studies, it appears that boys are highly susceptible to the modeling that is done when witnessing an adult or peer committing animal abuse. In fact, in Baldry's study, boys (67%) were two times more likely to commit animal abuse when compared to girls (34%). Witnessing peers commit animal cruelty and being a boy were the two variables most predictive of a subject committing animal abuse.

Clearly, the abuse of an animal by a child or adolescent is a warning sign for client functioning in that it can be indicative of the potential for violence against people (Kellert & Felthous, 1985). Children or adolescents who have committed school shootings and adult serial killers all have documented histories of animal abuse (Arkow, 1995; Fox, 1999). There are studies that acknowledge the connection between committing childhood animal abuse and subsequent aggressive crimes against people (Ascione, 1993, 2001, 2005; Miller & Knutson, 1997; Silverstein, Ascione & Kaufmann, 2004). When battered women were surveyed by Ascione (1998), 71% reported that their partner had either threatened or had actually hurt or killed at least one of the family companion animals. Many women report delaying leaving a violent home because of a threat to the family animals (Faver & Strand, 2003). Flynn (2000) stated that many of the battered women in his study identified their companion animal as an important source of emotional support for them. Most concerning, though, is how the act of animal abuse can be generationally transmitted through modeling. In the Ascione (1998) study, thirty-two percent of the battered women reported that one of their children had either physically harmed or killed one or more of the family pets. Therapists are well aware that cruelty toward animals is one criteria used in the diagnosis of conduct disorder (American Psychiatric Association, 2000). Recently, Dadds, Whiting, and Hawes (2006) identified that psychopathic traits, such as callousness or lack of emotionality, were strongly associated with committing animal abuse. The authors suggest that the act of animal abuse may be connected to a failure to develop empathy and conscience-driven behavior, which in turn could indicate future psychological difficulties.

It is important to note that a few authors are highlighting the notion that viewing children and adolescents as either victims or perpetrators of animal abuse limits the perspective of the role the human-animal relationship might play in homes where family violence is occurring (Barker, 1999; Barker, Barker, Dawson & Knisely, 1997; Erzinger, 2004; Nebbe, 1998). Barker et al. (1997) state that the sexual abuse survivors in their study often reported that their companion animal was their only friend at the time of their abuse. Erzinger (2004) suggests that companion animals help abused children cope with the family chaos and are powerful in their supportive role. Certainly, abuse survivors could receive the same physical and mental health benefits that have been identified in the literature addressing the benefits and healing aspects of the human-animal interaction (Schaefer, 2002).

CHARACTERISTICS OF ABUSED ANIMALS

There is more than the human victim that is involved in the experience of witnessing animal abuse, and one would be remiss to not mention the fact that the abused animal suffers greatly. Beyond loss of life, which is certainly an outcome that happens all too frequently, there are many different ways in which an animal can suffer maltreatment. The following behaviors have been identified and adapted from the work of several authors (Vermeulen & Odendall, 1993, cited in Patronek, 1998; Munro, 1998). An animal could be tortured, burned, shot at, poisoned, given drugs and alcohol, mutilated, drowned, suffocated/strangulated, sexually abused (bestiality), or be physically assaulted (hit with fist or other object, kicked, bitten, thrown, shaken). Like children and adolescents, animals can suffer from physical abuse as well as sexual abuse. Munro (1999) discusses case studies of a unique form of animal abuse, Munchausen syndrome by proxy, where the animal is repetitively injured and needing veterinary care. Animals can also suffer from physical or emotional neglect including being abandoned, deprived of food, water, shelter, necessary veterinary care to alleviate suffering from illness or injury, sanitation, or experience general neglect as reflected in a lack of bodily care and grooming. Finally, animals can be hoarded, exposed to dog or cock fighting, deprived of social contact, exposed to conditions whereby the animal does not thrive, not given necessary affection and attention, or be emotionally terrorized and/or isolated.

Because veterinarians are often the first professionals to come into contact with the abused companion animal, livestock or wildlife, guidelines have been established to help them recognize and identify such abuse and neglect. For example, the Tufts Animal Condition and Care (TACC) scales (Patronek, 1998) have been created to assist veterinarians and others in screening and determining whether or not an animal is experiencing chronic or acute neglect. The TACC scales provide guidance around assessing the body condition of the animal and include a weather safety scale to determine risk associated with exposure to extreme temperatures. The TACC scales also include an environmental health scale to determine the sanitation condition of the area or facility used to house the animal and a physical care scale to determine general care conditions (e.g., matted hair that restricts movement and/or vision, soiled coat, condition of nails, etc.).

DEFINING ANIMAL ABUSE
USING CHILD ABUSE TYPOLOGIES

Several authors have noted that parallels exist between the various forms of child abuse and neglect and the abuse and neglect an animal might experience. These authors have suggested using the same classification systems of physical abuse and neglect, sexual abuse, and emotional abuse and neglect when assessing animal abuse (Ascione, Kaufmann, & Brooks, 2000; Munro, 1999). Munro mentions that there are corresponding behaviors between animals and babies or young children, including the fact that neither can speak for themselves nor directly express any pain and suffering they may be experiencing. As a result, one is left to "read" the nonverbal behaviors that might indicate abuse is occurring, which leaves the door open for degrees of uncertainty in making such a diagnosis. In assessing whether or not an animal has been abused, Munro suggests that the veterinarian consider the following owner behaviors that might indicate that the animal is being battered or neglected: the account of the accident does not fit with the observed injury, the owner does not provide necessary information to determine how the injury occurred, the owner exhibits a lack of concern or empathy for the suffering of the animal, and/or there is a delay in obtaining veterinary care for the injured animal (p. 203).

Also paralleling child abuse, the behavioral signs that an abused animal might exhibit include aggressive behavior, particularly if it is a dog used in dog fights, being subdued, and/or frightened in the presence of their human companion but able to express freely their playfulness when the owner has left the room (Munro, 1999). Given that animals are unable to clearly communicate what is happening to them, one has to draw upon the most compelling information possible in confirming that animal abuse has indeed occurred. Obviously, behavioral signs would be considered to have lower probability (Faller, 1993) in the confirmation of abuse, particularly since animals, like children, often love their human companions and behaviorally might exhibit a strong desire to please and/or indicate happiness when interacting with their human companions even if they are being abused by them. Physical indicators would have higher levels of probability that abuse occurred (Faller, 1993). Clearly, the more indicators of abuse that a veterinarian can obtain, the more certain one can be in identifying abuse and neglect. The documentation of signs of cruelty and neglect is critical, and it is necessary for the veterinarian to complete thoroughly written medical records and attempt to photograph and/or videotape the animal's injuries and overall condition (Yoffe-Sharp & Sinclair, 1998).

IMPLICATIONS

What Is There to Gain from Healthy Relationships Between Animals and Humans?

One way of examining human relationships with nonhuman animals is to examine what occurs when the relationship is an abusive and hurtful one. What about the flip side of the coin; how might healthy relationships teach us about nonviolence? A number of authors have written about the therapeutic effects that can occur between humans and animals both in and out of the clinical setting (Beck, 2000; Beck & Katcher, 1996; Hines & Bustad, 1986; Levinson, 1962, 1969; Schaefer, 2002; Serpell, 2000). Although the data is correlational, it appears that our relationship with animals can enhance our physical health (Allen, Blascovich, & Mendes, 2002; Friedmann, Katcher, Lynch, & Thomas, 1980; Friedmann, 2000; Friedmann & Thomas, 1995; Siegel, 1993) as well as our psychological health by decreasing stress, anxiety, and levels of depression (Hart, 2000; Johnson, Garrity, & Stallones, 1992; Noonan, 1998; Wilson, 1994). Triebenbacher (2000) has described the various roles the companion animal plays in the family system, including providing a means to facilitate communication, defusing intense emotions, and serving as an "emotional barometer" of the family environment. The relationship between children, adolescents, and animals can be extremely powerful in a variety of ways. Both Melson (2001, 2003) and Ascione (2005) have eloquently described the various roles animals play in the lives of children, including teaching children about emotional regulation and "attunement," which refers to the perceptual awareness of self and other and bridging the two (Lasher, 1998). Companion animals also present an opportunity for children to learn how to express compassion, empathy, and nurturance to others. Boys have limited socially accepted ways of expressing empathy and nurturance, and their relationship to animals can provide such an experience. Companion animals can offer the child a sense of security, social and emotional support, opportunities to play, and a chance to have a confidant. Clearly, the relationship with animals can enhance a child's development and growth. It is important to note that a large number of treatment programs for delinquent or disturbed children, teens, and adults have developed that are based upon the healing relationship with animals (see Ross, 1999; Teumer, 2003).

Attention needs to be paid to the impact humans have on animals as well and whether or not the relationships are equally positive for the animal. Several studies have noted that animals can experience some of the similar positive effects as humans do when interacting together. Beck (2000) and Hama, Yogo, and Matsuyama (1996) report that dogs and horses have lower heart rates and blood pressures when a human is stroking them. Topál, Miklósi, Csányi, and Dóka (1998) discovered that similar to the secure base parents provide their children, dogs tend to spend more time playing and exploring their world in the presence of their human companions. When the dogs were removed from the owner for a period of time, upon return, the dog was physically closer to its human companion before being able to explore their world once again. Similar to humans, dogs need a sense of safety and security for healthy development as well.

RECOMMENDATIONS

First and foremost, it appears that education about the nature and importance of animal abuse is critical for both the general population as well as for therapists who work with those who witness (or are threatened) animal abuse. Therapists, similar to the veterinarians who treat abused animals, are in a unique position in that they may be one of the first professionals to encounter a report of animal abuse from a client who has either witnessed abuse or committed it. Aware of the impact animal abuse can have on the human and animal victims, therapists need to be willing to ask the hard questions about animal abuse in the initial interview as well as remain attentive to the issue throughout the course of therapy with a given client. It is important to note that several authors have mentioned that clients often do not voluntarily offer information that they have been a victim of abuse unless the therapist asks directly (Pruitt & Kappius, 1992; Read & Fraser, 1998). The same could hold true with clients not voluntarily reporting witnessing, being threatened with or forced to commit animal abuse (Schaefer, Hays, & Steiner, in press). Therapists might consider drawing upon the Boat Inventory on Animal-Related Experiences (Boat, 1999) for guidance on questions to ask regarding animal abuse.

Therapists need training in the therapeutic models for treating animal abusers such as the AniCare Model (Jory & Randour, 1999) if working with adult offenders or the AniCare Child (Randour et al., 2002) model of treatment if working with both witnesses of animal abuse and offending. These models draw upon an integration of cognitive-behavioral, social learning, psychodynamic and Gestalt theories. The treatment approach depicts a schematic of four layers, behavior, personal beliefs, family, and subculture, to understand the occurrence of the abusive behavior. Based upon these models, the clinical work with animal abuse offenders keys in on the development of empathy and becoming accountable for the abusive behavior and various exercises that are based upon seven concepts are used to facilitate the treatment process. Training in the two treatment models can be obtained by contacting Animals and Society Institute at http://www.animals andsociety.org/.

Assessing victims who witnessed animal abuse for post-traumatic stress symptoms and other "internalizing" and "externalizing" symptoms will be gravely important for therapists who work with victims. Because we know that many women do not leave abusive husbands due to the threats of cruelty that have been made against the family companion animals and livestock (Ascione, 1998, 2005; Flynn, 2000; Quinlisk, 1999), therapists need to ask battered women if this is one factor that may be holding them back from leaving. Therapists can also work to establish programs to assist domestic violence shelters in finding ways of fostering the animals so that a woman can leave the abusive environment (Jorgensen & Maloney, 1999). Increasingly, states are now addressing the connection between animal abuse and relationship violence. In April 2006, the state of Maine, in its recognition that animal abuse was stopping women from leaving violent homes, decided to include the family companion animals under any protection (restraining) order (Belluck, 2006).

A challenging situation pertaining to animal abuse can occur when a therapist encounters clients that are currently committing animal abuse. Different from child or vulnerable adult abuse, there are no state statutes that require therapists to break confidentiality in these situations in spite of the fact that there is clearly a relationship between animal abuse and human violence. Schaefer, Hays, and Steiner (2007) suggest that this is an issue needing to be addressed at the level of the therapists' professional association. In educating mental health professionals, ethical concerns, such as mandatory reporting of animal abuse, may arise, warranting discussion of how to ethically address this.

In order to disrupt the cycle of violence, it appears that all forms of family violence need to be addressed in order for change to occur. Animal abuse is one form of family violence that is just beginning to be acknowledged as a critical mental health and societal issue. It will be important for therapists to address animal abuse as it occurs in families and communities as well as be responsive to clients who report being a victim or perpetrator of animal abuse. Finally, there is an increasing need to assist the other professionals (for example, in the judicial system, state legislature, medical settings) who may come into contact with victims and abusers.

AUTHOR NOTE

Karen D. Schaefer received her PhD in counseling psychology from the University of Illinois at Urbana-Champaign. She is the training coordinator at New Mexico State University Counseling Center. In addition to training and supervision, her areas of professional interest include adult survivors of childhood abuse (physical, emotional, sexual, neglect) or trauma, grief and loss issues, offenders of abuse, animal abuse including offenders and victims who witnessed such abuse, the healing aspects of human-animal interactions and the provision of animal assisted therapy as an adjunct to psychotherapy.

REFERENCES

Allen, K. M., Blascovich, J., & Mendes, W.B. (2002). Cardiovascular reactivity and the presence of pets, friends, and spouses: The truth about cats and dogs. *Psychosomatic Medicine, 64,* 727-739.

American Humane Association. (2006). *Emotional abuse.* Retrieved January 11, 2007, from http://www.americanhumane.org/site/PageServer?pagename=nr_fact_sheets_child-emotion.

American Psychiatric Association. (2000). *Diagnostic and statistical manual of mental disorders* (4th ed., text rev.). Washington, DC: Author.

Arata, C. M., Langhinrichsen-Rohling, J., Bowers, D., & O'Farrill-Swails, L. (2005). Single versus multi-type maltreatment: An examination of the long-term effects of child abuse. *Journal of Aggression, Maltreatment & Trauma, 11*(4), 29-52.

Arkow, P. (1995). *Breaking the cycles of violence: A practical guide.* Alameda, CA: The Latham Foundation.

Arluke, A. (2002). Secondary victimization in companion animal abuse: The owner's perspective. In A. L. Podberscek, E. S., Paul, & J. A. Serpell (Eds), *Companion animals and us: Exploring the relations between people and pets* (pp. 275-291). Cambridge, UK: Cambridge University Press.

Ascione, F. R. (1993). Children who are cruel to animals: A review of research and implications for developmental psychopathology. *Anthrozoos, 6,* 226-247.

Ascione, F. R. (1998). Battered women's reports of their partners' and their children's cruelty to animals. *Journal of Emotional Abuse, 1*(1), 119-133.

Ascione, F. R. (2001, September). Animal abuse and youth violence. *Juvenile Justice Bulletin,* U.S. Department of Justice, Office of Juvenile Justice and Delinquency Prevention.

Ascione, F. R. (2005). *Children and animals: Exploring the roots of kindness and cruelty.* West Lafayette, IN: Purdue University Press.

Ascione, F. R., Friedrich, W. N., Heath, J., & Hayashi, K. (2003). Cruelty to animals in normative, sexually abused, and outpatient psychiatric samples of 6- to 12- year-old children: Relations to maltreatment and exposure to domestic violence. *Anthrozoos, 16*(3), 194-212.

Ascione, F. R., Kaufmann, M. E., & Brooks, S. M. (2000). Animal abuse and developmental psychopathology: Recent research, programmatic, and therapeutic issues and challenges for the future. In A. Fine (Ed.), *Handbook on animal-assisted therapy: Theoretical foundations and guidelines for practice* (pp. 325-354). New York: Academic Press.

Baker, D. G., Boat, B. W., Grinvalsky, H. T., & Geracioti, T. D. (1998). Interpersonal trauma and animal-related experiences in female and male military veterans: Implications for program development. *Military Medicine, 163,* 20-26.

Baldry, A. C. (2003). Animal abuse and exposure to interparental violence in Italian youth. *Journal of Interpersonal Violence, 19*(3), 258-281.

Barker, S. B. (1999). Therapeutic aspects of the human-companion animal interaction. *Psychiatric Times, 16,* 43-45. Retrieved January 5, 2007, from http://www.psychiatric times.com/p990243.html.

Barker, S. B., Barker, R. T., Dawson, K. S., & Knisely, J. S. (1997). The use of the family space diagram in establishing interconnectedness: A preliminary study of sexual abuse survivors, their significant others, and pets. *Individual Psychology, 53,* 435-450.

Beck, A. M. (2000). The use of animals to benefit humans: Animal-assisted therapy. In A. Fine (Ed.), *Handbook on animal-assisted therapy: Theoretical foundations and guidelines for practice* (pp. 21-40). New York: Academic Press.

Beck, A., & Katcher, A. (1996). *Between pets and people.* West Lafayette, IN: Purdue University Press.

Becker-Blease, K. A., & Freyd, J. J. (2005). Beyond PTSD: An evolving relationship between trauma theory and family violence research. *Journal of Interpersonal Violence, 20,* 403-411.

Belluck, P. (2006, April 1). New Maine law shields animals in domestic violence cases. *New York Times.* Retrieved April 4, 2006, from http://www.nytimes.com

Boat, B. W. (1999). Abuse of children and abuse of animals: Using the links to inform child assessment and protection. In F. R. Ascione & P. Arkow (Eds.), *Child abuse, domestic violence, and animal abuse: Linking the circles of compassion for prevention and intervention* (pp. 83-100). West Lafayette, IN: Purdue University Press.

Briere, J. N. & Elliott, D. M. (1994). Immediate and long-term impacts of child sexual abuse. *Future of Children, 4*(2), 54-69.

Conte, J. R., & Schuerman, J. R. (1987). Factors associated with an increased impact of child sexual abuse. *Child Abuse and Neglect, 11*(2), 201-211.

Cox, C. E., Kotch, J. B., & Everson, M. D. (2003). A longitudinal study of modifying influences in the relationship between domestic violence and child maltreatment. *Journal of Family Violence, 18*(1), 5-17.

Cunningham, A., & Baker, L. (2004). *What about me! Seeking to understand a child's view of violence in the family.* London: Centre for Children & Families in the Justice System.

Dadds, M. R., Whiting, C., & Hawes, D. J. (2006). Associations among cruelty to animals, family conflict, and psychopathic traits in childhood. *Journal of Interpersonal Violence, 21,* 411-429.

Davis, J. L., & Petretic-Jackson, P. A. (2000). The impact of child sexual abuse on adult interpersonal functioning: A review and synthesis of the empirical literature. *Aggression and Violent Behavior, 5*(3), 291-328.

DeRobertis, E. M. (2004). The impact of long-term psychological maltreatment by one's maternal figure: A study of the victim's perspective. *Journal of Emotional Abuse, 4*(2), 27-51.

Dinwiddie, S., Heath, A. C., Dunne, M. P., Bucholz, K. K., Madden, P. A., Slutske, W. S., et al. (2000). Early sexual abuse and lifetime psychopathology: A co-twin-control study. *Psychological Medicine, 30,* 41-52.

Dong, M., Anda, R. F., Dube, S. R., Giles, W. H., & Felitti, V .J. (2003). The relationship of exposure to childhood sexual abuse to other forms of abuse, neglect, and household dysfunction during childhood. *Child Abuse and Neglect, 27,* 625-639.

Dube, S. R., Anda, R. F., Whitfield, C. L., Brown, D. W., Felitti, V. J., Dong, M., et al. (2005). Long-term consequences of childhood sexual abuse by gender of victim. *American Journal of Preventative Medicine, 28*(5), 430-438.

Dutton, D. G. (2000). Witnessing parental violence as a traumatic experience shaping the abusive personality. *Journal of Aggression, Maltreatment and Trauma, 3*(1), 59-67.

Edleson, J. L. (1999). Children's witnessing of adult domestic violence. *Journal of Interpersonal Violence, 14,* 839-870.

Edwards, V. J., Holden, G. W., Felitti, V. J., & Anda, R. F. (2003). Relationship between multiple forms of childhood maltreatment and adult mental health in community respondents: Results from the adverse childhood experiences study. *American Journal of Psychiatry, 160*(8), 1453-1460.

Erzinger, S. (2004). Children in violent homes: How pets help them cope. *Protecting Children, 19*, 19-23.

Faller, K. C. (1993). *Child sexual abuse: Intervention and treatment issues.* McLean, VA: The Circle, Inc.

Famularo, R., Kinscherff, R., & Fenton, T. (1992). Psychiatric diagnoses of maltreated children: Preliminary findings. *Journal of the American Academy of Child and Adolescent Psychiatry, 31*, 863-867.

Faver, C. A., & Strand, E. B. (2003). To leave or to stay? Battered women's concern for vulnerable pets. *Journal of Interpersonal Violence, 18*, 1367-1377.

Flynn, C. P. (1999). Exploring the link between corporal punishment and children's cruelty to animals. *Journal of Marriage and the Family, 61*, 971-981.

Flynn, C. P. (2000). Woman's best friend: Pet abuse and the role of companion animals in the lives of battered women. *Violence Against Women, 6*, 162-177.

Fox, M. (1999). Treating serious animal abuse as a serious crime. In F. R. Ascione & P. Arkow (Eds.), *Child abuse, domestic violence, and animal abuse: Linking the circles of compassion for prevention and intervention* (pp. 306-315). West Lafayette, IN: Purdue University Press.

Friedmann, E. (2000). The animal-human bond: Health and wellness. In A. Fine (Ed.), *Handbook on animal-assisted therapy: Theoretical foundations and guidelines for practice* (pp. 41-58). New York: Academic Press.

Friedmann, E., Katcher, A. H., Lynch, J. J., & Thomas, S. A. (1980). Animal companions and one-year survival from a coronary care unit. *Public Health Reports, 95*(4), 307-312.

Friedmann, E., & Thomas, S. A. (1995). Pet ownership, social support, and one-year survival after acute myocardial infarction in the cardiac arrhythmia suppression trial (CAST). *American Journal of Cardiology, 76*, 1213-1217.

Garbarino, J., Guttman, E., & Seeley, J. (1986). *The psychologically battered child.* San Francisco: Jossey-Bass.

Graham-Bermann, S. A., & Hughes, H. M. (1998). The impact of domestic violence and emotional abuse on children: The intersection of research, theory, and clinical intervention. *Journal of Emotional Abuse, 1*(2), 1-21.

Graham-Bermann, S. A., & Levendosky, A. A. (1998). Traumatic stress symptoms in children of battered women. *Journal of Interpersonal Violence, 13*(1), 111-128.

Hama, H., Yogo, M., & Matsuyama, Y. (1996). Effects of stroking horses on both humans' and horses' heart rate responses. *Journal of Psychological Research, 38*(2), 66-73.

Hart, L. A. (2000). Psychosocial benefits of animal companionship. In A. H. Fine (Ed.), *Handbook on animal- assisted therapy: Theoretical foundations and guidelines for practice* (pp. 59-78). New York: Academic Press.

Herman, J. L. (1992). *Trauma and recovery.* New York: Basic Books.

Hines, L. M., & Bustad, L. K. (1986). Historical perspectives on human-animal interactions. *National Forum, 66*, 4-6.

Johnson, T. P., Garrity, T. F., & Stallones, L. (1992). Psychometric evaluation of the Lexington attachment to pets scale (LAPS). *Anthrozoös, 5*(3), 160-175.

Johnson, R. M., Kotch, J. B., Catellier, D. J., Winsor, J. R., Dufort, V., Hunter, W., et al. (2002). Adverse behavioral and emotional outcomes from child abuse and witnessed violence. *Child Maltreatment, 7*(3), 179-186.

Jorgensen, S., & Maloney, L. (1999). Animal abuse and the victims of domestic violence. In F. R. Ascione & P. Arkow (Eds.), *Child abuse, domestic violence, and animal abuse: Linking the circles of compassion for prevention and intervention* (pp. 143-158). West Lafayette, IN: Purdue University Press.

Jory, B., & Randour, M. L. (1999). *The AniCare model of treatment for animal abuse. Washington Grove, MD: Psychologists for the Ethical Treatment of Animals.*

Kellert, S. R., & Felthous, A. R. (1985). Childhood cruelty towards animals among criminals and noncriminals. *Human Relations, 38,* 1113-1129.

Kendler, K. S., Bulik, C. M., Silberg, J., Hettema, J. M., Myers, J., & Prescott, C. A. (2000). Childhood sexual abuse and adult psychiatric and substance use disorders in women: An epidemiological and co-twin control analysis. *Archives of General Psychiatry, 57,* 953-959.

Kerig, P. K., Fedorowicz, A. E., Brown, C. A., & Warren, M. (2000). Assessment and intervention for PTSD in children exposed to violence. *Journal of Aggression, Maltreatment & Trauma, 3*(1), 161-184.

Kilpatrick, K. L., Litt, M., & Williams, L. M. (1997). Posttraumatic stress disorder in child witnesses to domestic violence. *American Journal of Orthopsychiatry, 67*(4), 639-644.

Lansford, J. E., Dodge, K. A., Pettit, G. S., Bates, J. E., Crozier, J., & Kaplow, J. (2002). A 12-year prospective study of the long-term effects of early child physical maltreatment on psychological, behavioral, and academic problems in adolescence. *Archives of Pediatric Adolescent Medicine, 156,* 824-830.

Lasher, M. (1998). A relational approach to the human-animal bond. *Anthrozoös, 11*(3), 130-133.

Levinson, B. M. (1962). The dog as a "co-therapist." *Mental Hygiene, 46,* 59-65.

Levinson, B. M. (1969). *Pet-oriented child psychotherapy.* Springfield, IL: Charles C. Thomas, Publisher.

McFarlane, J. M., Groff, J. Y., O'Brien, J. A., & Watson, K. (2003). Behaviors of children who are exposed and not exposed to intimate partner violence: An analysis of 330 black, white, and Hispanic children. *Pediatrics, 112*(3), e202-e207.

McGuigan, W. M., & Middlemiss, W. (2005). Sexual abuse in childhood and interpersonal violence in adulthood: A cumulative impact on depressive symptoms in women. *Journal of Interpersonal Violence, 20*(10), 1271-1287.

Melson, G. F. (2001). *Why the wild things are: Animals in the lives of children.* Cambridge, MA: Harvard University Press.

Melson, G. F. (2003, May). *Animals in the lives of children.* Paper presented at the Delta Society 17th Annual Conference, Seattle, WA.

Miller, K. S., & Knutson, J. R. (1997). Reports of severe physical punishment and exposure to animal cruelty by inmates convicted of felonies and by university students. *Child Abuse and Neglect, 21,* 59-82.

Munro, H. M. C. (1998). The battered pet syndrome. In P. Olson (Ed.), *Recognizing and reporting animal abuse: A guide for veterinarians* (pp. 76-82). Englewood, CO: American Humane Association.

Munro, H. M. C. (1999). The battered pet. In F. R. Ascione & P. Arkow (Eds.), *Child abuse, domestic violence, and animal abuse: Linking the circles of compassion for prevention and intervention* (pp. 199-208). West Lafayette, IN: Purdue University Press.

Nebbe, L. (1998). *The human-animal bond's role with the abused child.* Paper presented at the Delta Society 17th Annual Conference, Seattle, WA.

Ney, P. G., Fung, T., & Wickett, A. R. (1994). The worst combinations of child abuse and neglect. *Child Abuse and Neglect, 18*, 705-714.

Noonan, E. (1998, May). People and pets. *Psychodynamic Counselling, 4*(1), 17-31.

Patronek, G. J. (1998). Issues and guidelines for veterinarians in recognizing, reporting, and assessing animal neglect and abuse. In P. Olson (Ed.), *Recognizing and reporting animal abuse: A guide for veterinarians* (pp. 25-39). Englewood, CO: American Humane Association.

Pruitt, J. A., & Kappius, R. E. (1992). Routine inquiry into sexual victimization: A survey of therapists' practices. *Professional Psychology: Research and Practice, 28*, 474-479.

Quinlisk, J. A. (1999). Animal abuse and family violence. In F. R. Ascione & P. Arkow (Eds.), *Child abuse, domestic violence, and animal abuse: Linking the circles of compassion for prevention and intervention* (pp. 168-175). West Lafayette, IN: Purdue University Press.

Randour, M. L., Krinsk, S., & Wolf, J. L. (2002). *AniCare child: An assessment and treatment approach for childhood animal abuse.* Washington Grove, MD: Psychologists for the Ethical Treatment of Animals.

Raupp, C. D., Barlow, M., & Oliver, J. A. (1997). Perceptions of family violence: Are companion animals in the picture? *Society and Animals, 5*, 219-238.

Read, J., & Fraser, A. (1998). Abuse histories of psychiatric inpatients: To ask or not to ask? *Psychiatric Services, 49*, 355-359.

Ross, S. B. (1999). Green chimneys: We give troubled children the gift of giving. In F. R. Ascione & P. Arkow (Eds.), *Child abuse, domestic violence, and animal abuse: Linking the circles of compassion for prevention and intervention* (pp. 367-379). West Lafayette, IN: Purdue University Press.

Runyon, M. K., & Kenny, M. C. (2002). Relationship of attributional style, depression, and posttrauma distress among children who suffered physical or sexual abuse. *Child Maltreatment, 7*(3), 254-264.

Schaefer, K. (2002). Human-animal interactions as a therapeutic intervention. *Counseling and Human Development, 34*(5), 1-18.

Schaefer, K. D., Hays, K. A., & Steiner, R. L. (2007). Animal abuse issues in therapy: A survey of therapists' attitudes. *Professional Psychology: Research and Practice, 38*(5), 530-537.

Serpell, J. A.(2000). Animal companions and human well-being: An historical exploration of the value of human-animal relationships. In A. H. Fine (Ed.), *Handbook on animal-assisted therapy: Theoretical foundations and guidelines for practice* (pp. 3-19). New York: Academic Press.

Siegel, J. M. (1993). Companion animals: In sickness and in health. *Journal of Social Issues, 49*(1), 157-167.

Silverstein, M., Ascione, F. R., & Kaufmann, M. E. (2004). Understanding the link between violence to people and animals: An indispensable tool for child welfare professionals. *Protecting Children, 19,* 2-3.

Spataro, J., Mullen, P. E., Burgess, P. M., Wells, D. L., & Moss, S. A. (2004). Impact of
child sexual abuse on mental health: Prospective study in males and females. *British
Journal of Psychiatry, 184,* 416-421.

Spertus, I. L, Yehuda, R., Wong, C. M., Halligan, S., & Seremetis, S. V. (2003). Childhood emotional abuse and neglect as predictors of psychological and physical
symptoms in women presenting to a primary care practice. *Child Abuse and Neglect, 27,* 1247-1258.

Steel, J., Sanna, L., Hammond, B., Whipple, J., & Cross, H. (2004). Psychological
sequelae of childhood sexual abuse: Abuse-related characteristics, coping strategies, and attributional style. *Child Abuse and Neglect, 28,* 785-801.

Swanston, H. Y., Plunkett, A. M., O'Toole, B. I., Shrimpton, S., Parkinson, P. N., &
Oates, R. K. (2003). Nine years after child sexual abuse. *Child Abuse and Neglect,
27,* 967-984.

Teumer, S. (2003, May). *Our farm program of experiential learning.* Paper presented
at the Delta Society 17th Annual Conference, Seattle, WA.

Topál, J., Miklósi, Á., Csányi, V., & Dóka, A. (1998). Attachment behavior in dogs
(*Canis familiaris*): A new application of Ainsworth's (1969) strange situation test.
Journal of Comparative Psychology, 112(3), 219-229.

Triebenbacher, S. L. (2000). The companion animal within the family system: The
manner in which animals enhance life within the home. In A. H. Fine (Ed.), *Handbook on animal- assisted therapy: Theoretical foundations and guidelines for practice* (pp. 357-374). New York: Academic Press.

Turkel, A., & Shaw, C. (2003). Domestic violence basics for child abuse professionals.
National Center for the Prosecution of Child Abuse Update Newsletter, 16(1), 1-5.

Turner, H. A., Finkelhor, D., & Ormrod, R. (2006). The effect of lifetime victimization
on the mental health of children and adolescents. *Social Science and Medicine,
62,*13-27.

Tyler, K. A. (2002). Social and emotional outcomes of childhood sexual abuse: A review of recent research. *Aggression and Violent Behavior, 7,* 567-589.

Valle, L. A., & Silovsky, J. F. (2002). Attributions and adjustment following child sexual abuse and physical abuse. *Child Maltreatment, 7*(1), 9-24.

Wilson, C. (1994). A conceptual framework for human-animal interaction research:
The challenge revisited. *Anthrozoös, 7*(1), 4-12.

Windom, C. S., DuMont, K., & Czaja, S. J. (2007). A prospective investigation of major depression in abused and neglected children grown up. *Archives of General Psychiatry, 64,* 49-56.

Yoffe-Sharp, B., & Sinclair, L. (1998). The veterinarian's role in investigating animal
cruelty. In P. Olson (Ed.), *Recognizing and reporting animal abuse: A guide for veterinarians,* (pp. 55-59). Englewood, CO: American Humane Association.

Ystgaard, M., Hestetun, I., Loeb, M., & Mehlum, L. (2004). Is there a specific relationship between childhood sexual and physical abuse and repeated suicidal behavior?
Child Abuse and Neglect, 28, 863-875.

doi:10.1300/J135v07n03_03

Animal Abuse and Domestic Violence: A View from the Border

Catherine A. Faver
Alonzo M. Cavazos, Jr.

SUMMARY. Previous research indicates that batterers often threaten or harm pets in order to intimidate and control their female partners. Most of this research, however, has been limited to samples comprised primarily of non-Hispanic women. To address this gap, this paper reports findings from a survey of 151 pet-owning women (74% Hispanic) who sought help from two South Texas domestic violence programs near the U.S.-Mexico border. Thirty-six percent of the women reported that their batterers had threatened, harmed, or killed their pets; 35% reported that they worried about the safety of their pets while they were in the abusive relationship; and 20.5% reported that concern for the safety of their pets affected their decision about seeking shelter. The findings indicate that pet abuse is a component of intimate partner violence (IPV) in Hispanic as well as non-Hispanic families. doi:10.1300/J135v07n03_04 *[Article copies available for a fee from The Haworth Document Delivery Service: 1-800-HAWORTH. E-mail address: <docdelivery@haworthpress.com> Website: <http://www.HaworthPress.com> © 2007 by The Haworth Press. All rights reserved.]*

Address correspondence to: Catherine A. Faver, PhD, LMSW, Department of Social Work at the University of Texas-Pan American, 1201 West University Drive, Edinburg, TX 78541 (E-mail: cfaver@utpa.edu).

[Haworth co-indexing entry note]: "Animal Abuse and Domestic Violence: A View from the Border." Faver, Catherine A., and Alonzo M. Cavazos, Jr. Co-published simultaneously in *Journal of Emotional Abuse* (The Haworth Maltreatment & Trauma Press, an imprint of The Haworth Press) Vol. 7, No. 3, 2007, pp. 59-81; and: *Animal Abuse and Family Violence: Linkages, Research, and Implications for Professional Practice* (ed: Marti T. Loring, Robert Geffner, and Janessa Marsh) The Haworth Maltreatment & Trauma Press, an imprint of The Haworth Press, 2007, pp. 59-81. Single or multiple copies of this article are available for a fee from The Haworth Document Delivery Service [1-800-HAWORTH, 9:00 a.m. - 5:00 p.m. (EST). E-mail address: docdelivery@haworthpress.com].

KEYWORDS. Emotional abuse, intimate partner violence, animal abuse, Hispanic women, Mexican-American women, Latinas

Previous research demonstrates that batterers often threaten or harm pets in order to intimidate, control, and coerce their female partners (Ascione, 1998; Faver & Strand, 2003a, b; Flynn, 2000a, b, c). Most of this research, however, has been limited to samples comprised primarily of non-Hispanic women. This limitation is important because the rate of pet ownership is lower among Hispanics than Anglos (Pew Research Center, 2006), and there is some evidence suggesting that attachment to pets may be linked to ethnicity as well (Siegel, 1995). To broaden our understanding of the co-occurrence of animal abuse and domestic violence, this paper reports findings from a sample of pet-owning women, the majority of whom are of Mexican descent, who sought help from two domestic violence programs in the Lower Rio Grande Valley of Texas.

This study replicated questions used in previous studies of animal abuse and domestic violence in order to determine whether rates of pet ownership and pet abuse were similar to those found in samples of non-Hispanic battered women. Specifically, the study asked: How common is pet ownership among women seeking help from two domestic violence programs near the Texas-Mexico border? What percentage of domestic violence clients in these two programs reported that their partners threatened or harmed their pets? To what extent were the women concerned about their pets, and did concern for their pets affect the women's decision about seeking shelter?

The demographic and social features of Texas's Lower Rio Grande Valley (LRGV) form the backdrop of this study. The LRGV includes four counties (Cameron, Willacy, Hidalgo, and Starr) in the southernmost part of Texas. The Rio Grande River, which forms the U.S.-Mexico border, is the southern border of three of the four counties (Cameron, Hidalgo, and Starr). The LRGV has a predominantly Hispanic population and a high poverty rate. The impact of these factors will be considered in reviewing several areas of knowledge relevant to this study: (a) the factors associated with domestic violence in Latino families, (b) pet abuse as a component of emotional abuse in the context of domestic violence, and (c) variations in pet ownership and attachment to pets related to ethnicity and social class.

Before proceeding, a note about terminology is in order. Because the study described in this paper was conducted near the U.S. border with

Mexico, most of the respondents were women of Mexican descent (either Mexican Americans or Mexican nationals residing in the U.S.). These women are a subgroup of the population generally referred to as Latinas or Hispanic women. Members of this ethnic group vary in their preferences about which term to use to identify their ethnicity. In reviewing the literature, this paper will use the terminology of the authors who are cited. Respondents in the current study will be described as "Mexican Americans and Mexican nationals," or as "Hispanic," which was the term used in the study questionnaire.

REVIEW OF THE LITERATURE

Latinas and Intimate Partner Violence

This study is based on feminist and sociological perspectives on intimate partner violence (IPV). A feminist perspective assumes that intimate partner violence is a reflection of gender oppression in a patriarchal society (Yllo, 1993). Specifically, batterers use both physical violence and emotional abuse to assert power and maintain control over women in intimate relationships (Adams, 1995; Flynn, 2000a, b, c). In addition, ethnicity, gender, and social class are not simply characteristics of individuals; these demographic factors are embedded in the social structure and manifested in differential privileges and penalties for members of dominant and subordinate groups (Andersen & Collins, 1998). Thus, the nature and consequences of IPV vary among women of different ethnic groups and social classes. As Yoshihama (2000) notes, "individuals' experiences of domestic violence must be understood in their unique socio-cultural contexts" (p. 208). Yet, there is relatively little research on Latinas' experience of domestic violence, and even fewer studies focusing specifically on Mexican Americans and Mexican nationals residing in the United States.

The studies examining ethnic group differences in rates of intimate partner violence have yielded conflicting findings regarding the rate of IPV among Latinas compared to White non-Hispanic women. Straus and Smith (1990) reported higher rates of IPV among Hispanics compared to non-Hispanic whites, while several other studies reported lower rates for Hispanics (Bachman, 1994; McFarlane, Parker, Koeken, & Bullock, 1992; Sorenson, Upchurch, & Shen, 1996). Moreover, several studies based on probability samples found no differences in rates of IPV among Hispanics and non-Hispanic whites (Kantor, Jasinski, &

Aldarondo, 1994; Neff, Holamon, & Schluter, 1995; Tjaden & Thoennes, 1998).

A second area of research focuses on risk factors for abuse and the correlates of IPV. Several studies have shown a positive relationship between increased acculturation to the U.S. and incidences of IPV (Sorenson & Telles, 1991; Kantor et al., 1994; Lown & Vega, 2001). Place of birth (U.S.-born or foreign-born) has often been used as an indicator of acculturation. Two studies (Kantor et al.; Sorenson & Telles) on perpetration of IPV by U.S. Hispanics, one of which focused specifically on Mexican Americans (Sorenson & Telles), found higher rates of IPV perpetrated by men born in the U.S. than among those born outside the U.S. Lown and Vega's study of Mexican American women found that U.S. birthplace was associated with IPV victimization, even after controlling for other factors commonly associated with IPV among both Hispanics and Anglos, including young age, urban residence, social isolation, and large number of children.

Lown and Vega (2001) also found that measures of acculturation other than place of birth, including length of time in the U.S., country of schooling, and a language-based acculturation scale, consistently showed a positive association between greater acculturation and IPV victimization. Although the preponderance of the evidence indicates a positive association between acculturation and IPV rates, one study differs slightly from the others. Specifically, Caetano, Schafer, Clark, Cunradi, and Raspberry (2000) found that moderately acculturated Hispanic men had the highest rates of perpetration of IPV, followed by highly acculturated men.

Level of acculturation is also related to help-seeking by Latina victims of domestic violence. Using data from a national sample, West, Kantor, and Jasinski (1998) found that Anglo victims of domestic violence were more likely than Latina victims to seek help. Moreover, within the sample of Latinas, level of acculturation, as measured by English language preference, was positively related to help-seeking. In other words, preference for speaking Spanish was a barrier to help-seeking.

Immigration status is another factor that affects Latinas' vulnerability to abuse and the likelihood that they will seek help. Victims of crime, including battered women, are entitled to police protection regardless of their immigration status, and law enforcement officers are not authorized to inquire about or report information about the victim's immigration status (Texas Council on Family Violence, 2005). Nevertheless, undocumented women fear deportation and are often socially isolated. Their abusers may threaten to have them deported, and the women may have limited access to accurate information about their legal rights. Thus, undocumented women often distrust the police and service providers and may be reluctant to seek help (Lie & Lowery, 2003; Rasche, 2000).

Some scholars have suggested that gender ideology within Latino culture, which reinforces a patriarchal family structure, increases Latinas' risk of victimization (Morash, Bui, and Santiago, 2000). For example, the idea of *familism* is often interpreted in a way that includes the expectation that a woman should remain with her husband even if he abuses her (Vasquez, 1994; see also Falicov, 1998).

In general, scholars focusing on the experiences of women of color have suggested that gendered role expectations that include acceptance of male authority may shape women's response to abuse and deter them from resisting and reporting their victimization (Kanuha, 1994; see also Yoshihama, 2000). For example, in a study of 129 women of Japanese descent in Los Angeles County who had been in abusive relationships, Yoshihama (2000) found that the women's internalization of the cultural value of male domination and female subordination was expressed in the women's suppression of their own needs. Moreover, Yoshihama noted that Japanese cultural values, including deference to male authority, persisted across generations regardless of acculturation and exerted a strong effect particularly in intimate relationships. Among Hispanics in the U.S., the persistence of the cultural value of male domination despite changes in actual family roles and responsibilities could create tension and help to explain why several studies cited earlier (e.g., Lown & Vega, 2001; Kantor et al., 1994) found a positive relationship between acculturation and incidences of IPV.

Based on their qualitative research, Morash et al. (2000) suggested that Mexican American women's risk of victimization increases when economic conditions make it difficult for men to find adequate employment, and women become the family breadwinners through access to low-paying jobs. In response to a reversal of traditional gender roles, men may attempt to reassert their dominant position in the family through violence. On the other hand, in their study of Mexican American women in California, Lown and Vega (2001) found that a male partner's unemployment and a woman's higher income relative to her partner's were not associated with the incidence of IPV. Thus, in considering the impact of Latino culture on the occurrence of IPV, it is important to note that culture is interpreted differently in different social environments (see Ramos & Carlson, 2004).

A history of institutional oppression and discrimination is a socio-cultural factor that affects how women of color respond to their victimization (Kanuha, 1994; Rasche, 2000; Yoshihama, 2000). In some cases, women of color remain silent about their abuse to protect their ethnic group from additional stigma, stereotyping, and discrimination (Kanuha, 1994). For example, like African American women (Sorenson, 1996), Latinas in many regions in the U.S. may be reluctant to call the police to respond to an episode of violence because they are afraid their partners will be discriminated against in the criminal justice system (Rasche, 2000). In the Texas-Mexico border region, where the population (including the police) is predominantly Hispanic, a battered woman may be fearful not because of her ethnicity but because of her own or her partner's immigration status if either is undocumented. In short, while all women of color experience oppression, the specific socio-cultural context must be considered to understand the precise impact of oppression and institutional discrimination on a woman's response to IPV.

Very little research has focused on the mental health consequences of IPV for Latinas. In a study of English-speaking Latinas varying in national origin, Ramos and Carlson (2004) found higher levels of anxiety, depression, and somatization among women who had experienced recent emotional abuse. These findings resonate with a study (Hampton & Gelles, 1994) showing that Black women's symptoms of psychological distress were positively associated with experiences of physical violence from their partners. Future research on Latinas should investigate the mental health consequences of both physical and emotional forms of IPV.

Pet Abuse and Intimate Partner Violence

As noted in the introduction, research on the link between pet abuse and family violence has utilized samples comprised primarily of non-Hispanic women. This limitation aside, five findings from previous studies are especially pertinent to the current investigation:

1. Pet ownership is common among battered women. Indeed, surveys of battered women in domestic violence shelters found that the percentage of pet owners ranged from 40% (Flynn, 2000c) to 92% (Ascione, Weber, & Wood, 1997). Given the high rates of pet ownership among battered women, it is important to examine the co-occurrence of pet abuse and other forms of family violence

and to determine the impact of pet abuse on all family members, including the pet.

2. Pet abuse is common in families where there is domestic violence. In studies of pet-owning female victims of domestic violence, the percentage of women who reported that their batterers abused the women's pets ranges from 46.5% (Flynn, 2000c) to 86% (Strand, 2003). A batterer's pet abuse affects children in the family as well. Upon witnessing pet abuse, some children imitate the abuse while others attempt to protect their pets from abuse (Ascione, 1998; Ascione et al., 1997; Quinlisk, 1999). For example, in Quinlisk's survey of 49 battered women whose partners had abused their pets, 76% of the women reported that their children had witnessed the abuse, and 54% of the children who witnessed the pet abuse imitated the behavior. In a study involving interviews with 39 children of battered women whose pets were abused, Ascione et al. (1997) found that 67% of the children saw or heard their pets being abused. While 51% of the children reported that they tried to protect their pets, 13% reported that they themselves had also hurt their pets.

3. Pets are an important source of emotional support for battered women. In a study of pet-owning women in a domestic violence shelter in South Carolina, 55% of women whose pets had been abused compared to 38.1% of those whose pets had not been abused reported that their pets were an important source of emotional support (Flynn, 2000c). Flynn speculated that the closer a woman feels to her pets, the more likely it is that the batterer will abuse the pets because the batterer's goal is to hurt the woman.

4. Research on pet-owning battered women also shows that the percentage of women who reported that they worried about the safety of their pets when they were in the abusive relationship ranged from 18% (Ascione, 1998) to 91% (Strand & Faver, 2005). Moreover, many women continued to worry about their pets after they left the abusive relationship, especially if their pets had been abused. For example, Flynn (2000c) found that 40% of pet-owning women continued to worry about their pets after coming into a shelter. However, 65% of those whose pets had been abused, compared to 15% of those whose pets had not been abused, continued to worry about their pets.

5. In previous studies the percentage of battered women who reported that concern for the safety of their pets affected their decision-making about staying with or leaving an abusive partner

ranged from 18% (Ascione, 1998) to 60% (Strand, 2003). In some cases, pet abuse was one of the factors that *prompted* a woman to leave her abusive partner (Strand, 2003). In most instances, however, women *delayed* leaving because (a) they could not take their pets with them, (b) they had no alternative safe place for their pets, and (c) they were afraid to leave their pets with the abuser (Flynn, 2000c; Ascione, 1998). In order to remove concern for pets as a barrier to women's departure from an abusive partner, many domestic violence agencies and anti-violence community coalitions have created "safe pet" programs to provide shelter for the pets of battered women (Ascione, 2000; Faver & Strand, in press).

Family Violence, Poverty, and Pets: The Study Context

The review thus far has focused on what is known about domestic violence among Hispanics in the U.S. nationwide and on the link between pet abuse and domestic violence among non-Hispanic samples included in previous research. As a context for this study, it is useful to examine the prevalence of domestic violence in Texas, the socioeconomic conditions that shape the lives of people in the Rio Grande Valley, and the factors associated with pet ownership.

In 2002 the Texas Council on Family Violence (TCFV) commissioned a statewide survey, based on probability sampling methods, to determine the prevalence of domestic violence in Texas (TCFV, 2003). The survey instrument defined "severe abuse" as having experienced at least one of the following types of abuse: physical abuse (such as hitting, choking, or slapping), sexual abuse, or having oneself or one's family threatened by a spouse or dating partner. Estimates based on the survey findings indicated that 31% of all Texans (including both men and women) have been severely abused at some point in their lives. Not surprisingly, women (all ethnic groups combined) reported higher rates of severe abuse than men. Over a fourth (27%) of women reported physical abuse, 14% reported forced sex, and 20% reported threats to themselves or their families (TCFV, 2003).

The survey findings also indicated that 39% of all Hispanic women reported having experienced severe abuse (TCFV, 2006). Unfortunately, the survey report did not include information on the percentages of Hispanic women who experienced each of the different forms of severe abuse (physical, sexual, and threats). Moreover, the survey report did not compare the rates of severe abuse for Hispanic and Anglo women.

As mentioned earlier, the Lower Rio Grande Valley has a predominantly Hispanic population and a high poverty rate. Table 1 shows population estimates, percentage of Hispanics, and percentage of the population living below the poverty line for the cities of Brownsville and Harlingen, where the domestic violence agencies in this study are located; for Cameron and Willacy Counties, which are served by these agencies; and for the state of Texas as a whole (U.S. Census Bureau, 2006). As the table indicates, Hispanics comprise 32% of the population of Texas, but they are approximately 85% of the population in Cameron and Willacy counties. Moreover, the poverty rate in Cameron and Willacy counties (33%) is more than twice the poverty rate for the state as a whole (15%).

A survey conducted by the Pew Research Center in 2005 provides the only national data on ethnicity and pet ownership (Pew Research Center, 2006). The Pew data indicated that 64% of white, non-Hispanic individuals, compared to 39% of Hispanics and 30% of Blacks, were pet owners at the time of the survey.

In addition to ethnicity, pet ownership is related to family size and income (American Veterinary Medical Association [AVMA], 2002; Pew Research Center, 2006). According to a survey conducted by the AVMA in 2001, 71.6% of couples and 68.9% of families with children were pet owners, while only 39.5% of single individuals were pet owners (AVMA, 2002). Both the Pew and AVMA surveys indicated that higher income people are more likely to own pets (AVMA, 2002; Pew Research Center, 2006). At least 60% of people with incomes of $30,000 and higher were pet owners, while only 45% of people with incomes less than $30,000 owned pets (Pew Research Center, 2006).

No information is available on pet ownership among Hispanics in the Rio Grande Valley. However, in light of the high poverty rate in the area, it is reasonable to speculate that the rate of pet ownership would be relatively low among women seeking domestic violence services in the Texas-Mexico border region. At the same time, it is important to note that "pet ownership" may be defined differently depending on the social context. For example, there are numerous stray cats and dogs in many low-income neighborhoods in the Rio Grande Valley. It is possible that some families care for stray animals and become attached to them, even though the families cannot afford veterinary care and may not try to prevent the animals from roaming the neighborhood. Clearly, it is a woman's (or her children's) attachment to an animal, regardless of whether the animal is "owned," that often makes the animal a target of abuse by a batterer.

TABLE 1. Population Size, Percent Hispanic, and Percent Below Poverty in Texas and Geographic Areas Served by Agencies in the Study

Location	Population[a]	% Hispanic[b]	% Below Poverty[c]
Cameron County	371,825	84.3%	33.1%
Brownsville	156,178	91.3%	36.0%
Harlingen	60,769	72.8%	24.9%
Willacy County	20,231	85.7%	33.2%
Texas	22,490,022	32.0%	15.4%

Note. The data were obtained from the U.S. Census Bureau (2006). The two domestic violence agencies serve Cameron County and one serves part of Willacy County.
[a]State and county estimates from 2004; city estimates from 2003
[b]Based on estimates from 2000
[c]Based on estimates from 1999

Relatively few studies have examined ethnic group differences in attitudes and practices related to pets. Siegel (1995) found that non-Hispanic White adolescents scored significantly higher than Latino adolescents on a measure of how important their pets were to them. This finding has not been replicated, however, and more recent research seems to challenge the notion of ethnic group differences in attachment to pets.

For example, a telephone survey of 368 pet owners in a county in the southwest region of the United States (Risley-Curtiss, Holley, & Wolf, 2006) revealed that Hispanics in the sample ($n = 41$) were less likely than members of other ethnic groups to own cats, to have a veterinarian for their pet, and to have had their pet spayed or neutered. In addition, in response to a question about what their pet offered them, Hispanics were more likely than members of other ethnic groups to indicate that they received a sense of personal safety from their pet. At the same time, there were no significant differences between Hispanics and members of other ethnic groups in the percentage reporting that they received emotional support, unconditional love, and companionship from their pets, and in the percentage agreeing with the statement, "My pet is a member of my family." Moreover, Johnson and Meadows (2002) reported that 79% of a small sample (*n* = 24) of Latinos aged 50 and older regarded their dogs as members of the family. Finally, a qualitative study of 15 women of color (Risley-Curtiss et al., 2006), including 9 women who were members of Hispanic subgroups, indicated that 13 of the women regarded their pets as family members. Thus, in light of research suggesting that Hispanics are likely to regard their pets as family members, it is reasonable to assume that male batterers in Hispanic families would also be likely to use pet abuse as a strategy to control their female partners.

Research Questions

In light of previous research, this study focused on five questions about Hispanic women seeking help from two domestic violence agencies in the LRGV. Specifically, the study asked:

1. How common is pet ownership?
2. What percentage of the women report that their batterers threatened, harmed, or killed their pets? What percentage of the women report that their children threatened, harmed, or killed their pets?
3. What percentage of the women report that their pets were an important source of emotional support during the abusive relationship?
4. What percentage of the women report that they were concerned about the safety of their pets during the abusive relationship?
5. What percentage of the women report that concern for the safety of their pets affected their decision about staying with or leaving their abusive partner?

METHOD

Sample

A total of 501 women were surveyed by staff members of two domestic violence agencies during the study period. The staff members who administered the "Pet Survey" recorded the ethnicity of the participants by checking one of the following options listed on the survey instrument: (a) *Hispanic*, (b) *White, Non-Hispanic*, (c) *African American*, (d) *American Indian*, (e) *Asian American*, or (f) *Other (specify)*. Frequencies and percentages for ethnicity by pet ownership appear in Table 2.

Of the 501 women surveyed, 68% were identified as Hispanic, and 8% were identified as White, Non-Hispanic. Less than 2% were classified as Other, and the ethnicity of almost 23% of the participants was not recorded.

Survey respondents were initially divided into two categories: pet owners and non pet owners. Almost one-third (32.95%) of the 501 respondents were pet owners. Of the Hispanic women in the sample, 33% were pet owners, while 55% of the non-Hispanic White women were pet owners (χ^2 (3) = 10.68, p = .014).

Within the group of pet owners (n = 165), 14 survey participants did not respond to pet abuse survey items that were the focus of the study. Thus, these surveys were not included in the analyses. As a result, the final sample of pet owners was 151. However, the actual sample size for some analyses is less than 151 because of missing data on some completed surveys and because some questionnaire items relevant to the research questions in this study were included only on the 12-item version of the "Pet Survey." Of the total sample of 151, 59% of the respondents completed the 12-item version of the survey instrument, which was administered to resident (in-shelter) clients in the two domestic violence agencies; 41% of the respondents completed the 9-item version of the "Pet Survey," which was administered to non-resident (advocacy and counseling) clients of the two domestic violence agencies where data was collected.

Of the 151 women in the study sample, 74% were Hispanic and 14% were non-Hispanic Whites. Two women (1%) were classified as other, and the ethnic identity of 17 women (11%) was not reported.

The median age of the women in the study sample was 31 years old (SD = 9.22), with a minimum age of 17 and a maximum age of 59. Sixty-five percent of the women reported that they had children under 18 years old while in the abusive relationship; 28% reported not having children under 18 years old; and no information about the presence of children was reported by 7% of the respondents.

Measures

A 9-item version and a 12-item version of the "Pet Survey" were created by adapting and modifying the "Pet Abuse Survey" (Strand, 2003; Strand & Faver, 2005). Pet ownership was assessed with two questions: (1) "Have you ever had pets in this relationship?" and (2) "Do you currently have any pets?" The response alternatives for each question were

TABLE 2. Ethnicity for Study Sample by Pet Ownership

	Ethnicity ($N = 501$)			
		White, Non-		
Pet Ownership	Hispanic	Hispanic	Other	No Response
	f (%)	f (%)	f (%)	f (%)
Own Pets	111 (32.7)	21 (55.3)	2 (25)	31 (26.96)
No Pets	229 (67.3)	17 (44.7)	6 (75)	84 (73.04)
Total	340	38	8	115
% of sample	67.86%	7.59%	1.60%	22.95

Note. Ethnicity data were not obtained for 115 respondents (22.95%).

(a) *yes* and (b) *no*. Pet abuse by partner was measured with the following question: "Has your partner ever threatened to harm your pet(s), actually harmed your pet(s), or killed your pet(s)?" Pet abuse by the respondent's children was measured with the following question: "Has your child ever threatened to harm your pet(s), actually harmed your pet(s), or killed your pet(s)?" For each of these questions, the respondent was asked to check all of the following response alternatives that applied: (a) *threatened to harm your pet(s)*, (b) *actually harmed your pet(s)*, (c) *killed your pet(s)*, and (d) *none of these.*

Concern for pets was measured with the following question: "In the relationship with your abuser, have you worried about the safety of your pet(s)?" The response alternatives were (a) *yes* and (b) *no*. The 12-item version of the questionnaire included the following question to assess the extent to which the respondent perceived her pet as a source of emotional support: "In dealing with the abuse you have experienced in this relationship, how important has your pet been as a source of emotional support?" The response alternatives were (a) *very important*, (b) *somewhat important*, and (c) *not at all important.*

In the 9-item version of the instrument administered to non-resident clients, the impact of concern for pets on the woman's decision-making was assessed with the following question: "Has concern over the safety of your pet(s) ever affected your decision about seeking shelter?" In the 12-item version of the instrument administered to resident (shelter) clients, the question was worded slightly differently: "Did concern over the safety of your pet(s) affect your decision to seek shelter?" The response alternatives for both versions of this question were (a) *no*, (b) *yes–delayed my seeking shelter*, and (c) *yes–prompted me to seek shelter*.

Data Collection

The data were collected during a one-year period (2004) at a domestic violence agency in Brownsville, Texas, and during a two and a half year period (Spring 2003–Fall 2005) at a domestic violence agency in Harlingen, Texas. The Brownsville agency, which serves southern Cameron County, yielded 15% of the survey respondents (22 of 151). Overall, including adults and children, the Brownsville agency served 450 resident clients and 901 non-resident clients during 2004. The Harlingen agency, which serves northern Cameron County and part of an adjacent county (Willacy), yielded 85% of the respondents (129 of 151). Overall, including adults and children, the Harlingen agency served 453 resident and 454 non-resident clients in 2004; in 2005, the Harlingen agency served 500 resident clients and 665 non-resident clients. As Table 1 indicates, the city of Brownsville, which is situated directly across the Rio Grande River from the city of Matamoros in Mexico, is about two and a half times larger than Harlingen and has a higher percentage of Hispanics (91% versus 73%) and a higher poverty rate (36% versus 25%).

During the study period, staff members from the two domestic violence agencies administered either the 9-item or 12-item version of the "Pet Survey" to 501 women who requested resident (shelter) or non-resident (advocacy or counseling) services. The surveys were administered during the intake process or during the period of residence at the shelter. The 9-item version of the "Pet Survey" was administered to non-resident clients and the 12-item version of the "Pet Survey" was administered to resident clients. Both forms were available in English and Spanish, but only 6% of the questionnaires in the sample of pet owners were completed in Spanish.

Two factors may account for the low percentage of questionnaires completed in Spanish. First, 85% of the participants were surveyed at the Harlingen agency. As Table 2 shows, Harlingen's population is 72.8% Hispanic, while Brownsville's population is 91.3% Hispanic. Because Harlingen has a higher percentage of Anglos than Brownsville, Hispanics in Harlingen are more likely to be English-speaking and they are likely to be more highly acculturated. Second, previous research indicates that Latinas who seek help for domestic violence problems are more highly acculturated than those who do not seek help (West et al., 1998); thus, the respondents in this study, who were seeking help for domestic violence, are likely to be among the more highly acculturated who speak English.

Data Analysis

Frequency distributions and descriptive statistics were computed for all variables. Bivariate tables were constructed to examine relationships between variables, and chi-square analyses were used to determine the statistical significance of bivariate relationships.

The rates of pet ownership and partners' pet abuse were computed for the sample as a whole and separately for Hispanic women and non-Hispanic women. Other analyses were conducted without distinctions between ethnic groups because of the relatively small proportion of non-Hispanic White women (14%) in the sample of 151 pet owners and because ethnicity was not recorded for 11% of the sample.

RESULTS

Pet Ownership and Abuse

In the total sample of pet owners, 98% of the women reported having pets while in the abusive relationship, and 72% reported currently having a pet. Of the 151 pet-owning women, 36% reported that their partners threatened, harmed, or killed their pets. Among these types of abuse, 6% reported that their partners had killed their pets. Considering ethnicity, 52.4% (11 of 21) of the White non-Hispanic women, compared to 32.4% (36 of 111) of the Hispanic women, reported that their partners abused their pets ($\chi^2(1) = 3.069$, NS).

Only the women who sought shelter services ($n = 89$) were asked whether their children threatened, harmed, or killed family pets. Of the

75 women who responded to this question, four percent (3 of 75) reported that a child had threatened, harmed, or killed a pet.

Pets as Emotional Support

Only the 12-item version of the Pet Survey, administered to resident (in-shelter) clients, included the question about how important pets had been as a source of emotional support during the woman's relationship with her abusive partner. In response, 62% (53 of 85) of the women reported that their pets were *very important* as a source of emotional support, and 38% (32 of 85) reported that their pets were *somewhat* or *not at all important* as a source of emotional support. Moreover, 88% (23 of 26) of those whose pets had been abused, compared to 51% (30 of 59) of those whose pets had not been abused, reported that their pets had been *very important* as a source of emotional support during the abusive relationship ($\chi^2(1) = 10.88$, $p < .001$).

Concern for Pets

Of the 151 pet-owning women, 35% reported that they worried about the safety of their pets while in the abusive relationship. However, women whose pets had been abused were more likely to report that they worried about the safety of their pets while in the abusive relationship ($\chi^2(1) = 91.73$, $p < .001$). Specifically, 87% (46 of 53) of the women whose pets had been abused, compared to only 7% (7 of 93) of the women whose pets had not been abused, reported that they worried about the safety of their pets while in the abusive relationship.

Decision-Making

Considering all pet-owning women, 20.5% (28 of 136) reported that concern for their pets affected their decision about seeking shelter (15 women did not respond to this question). Of the 28 women whose decision-making was affected by concern for pets, 26 reported that they delayed seeking shelter while two reported that concern for pets prompted them to seek shelter. If the sample is limited to women who reported that they worried about the safety of their pets while they were in the abusive relationship, 37% (19 of 51) reported that concern for pets affected their decision about seeking shelter.

DISCUSSION

Significance of the Findings

This is the first study to document the link between animal abuse and domestic violence in a sample of Hispanic women. Almost a third (32.4%) of pet-owning Hispanic women in the sample reported that their partners threatened, harmed, or killed their pets. Thus, as is true in other regions and population groups, pet abuse is used to intimidate and coerce women of Mexican descent living in the impoverished border region of south Texas.

In the sample of pet owners as a whole, the findings indicated that women whose pets had been abused were more likely to report that their pets were an important source of emotional support and that they were concerned about their pets during the abusive relationship. Moreover, over a third (37%) of the women who worried about their pets during the abusive relationship reported that concern for their pets affected their decision about seeking shelter. These findings are consistent with previous research (Flynn, 2000a) suggesting that a woman's attachment to her pet makes the pet an attractive target for a batterer who is trying to hurt a woman emotionally or prevent her from leaving the relationship (see also Adams, 1995).

This study did not investigate whether the respondents' children witnessed pet abuse, and only "in-shelter" respondents were asked whether their children had perpetrated pet abuse. Of the women who responded to this question, only 4% reported that their children had threatened, hurt, or killed family pets. This finding differs from previous research (Ascione et al., 1997; Quinlisk, 1999), which found higher rates of pet abuse perpetrated by children of domestic violence survivors. It is possible, however, that the respondents in the current study underreported the extent of animal abuse perpetrated by their children. Indeed, some researchers have suggested that the extent of children's abuse of animals may be underestimated because it is often not witnessed by parents and other adults (see Ascione, 2005).

Implications for Practice

Recognition of the link between animal cruelty and family violence has important implications for service providers and policy-makers. Indeed, during the past decade national organizations such as the Humane Society of the United States (HSUS) have focused on "the link" through national campaigns to raise public awareness, provide training and resources for volunteers and service providers, and facilitate coordinated community initiatives to prevent and end violence toward people and animals (see HSUS, 2006).

Several recommendations for practice should be emphasized in light of the current study. First, domestic violence agencies should include questions about pets and pet abuse in intake interviews and clinical assessments. Clients should be asked about the presence of animals in the family, whether any of their animals have been hurt, and if so, how this happened. Interviewers also need to help clients include family pets in their safety plans. Second, at the organizational level, domestic violence agencies must work with animal welfare organizations to provide "safe pet" programs to care for the animals of pet-owning women who wish to leave their abusive partners and have no alternative housing arrangements for their companion animals. Third, at the community level, domestic violence agencies must work with other human services providers, animal welfare professionals, law enforcement agencies, attorneys, judges, school personnel, and community volunteers to establish anti-violence coalitions. Such coalitions can help to establish "safe pet" programs, cross-train animal welfare and human services professionals, educate the public about the link between animal abuse and interpersonal violence, instigate humane education programs in schools, advocate for the establishment and enforcement of strong animal anti-cruelty laws, and establish treatment programs for abusers. For a more thorough discussion of these and other recommendations for practice and policy, see Faver and Strand (in press).

This study of Hispanic women serves as a reminder that these recommendations for practice must be implemented in ways that are sensitive to the cultural and economic context. For example, when questions about pets are added to an intake questionnaire, they must be translated into Spanish. Similarly, brochures about safety planning must include information about pets and must be available in Spanish. When inquiring about pets, domestic violence workers must be aware that a woman or her children may have formed a bond with a stray animal even though the family may not be able to afford veterinary care. If the client or her children are attached to the pet, the pet's well being must be considered in safety planning.

Limitations of the Study

Measurement. The questionnaire items used in this study were adapted from instruments used in prior research; thus, this investigation shares the measurement limitations of previous studies. To begin, the questions on pet ownership and pet abuse required respondents to rely on their own definitions of these concepts, which may vary considerably among respondents. As noted earlier, some low-income Hispanic families may provide intermittent or continuous care for a stray animal without necessarily perceiving the animal as their "pet." If women who care for stray animals replied "no" to the question of whether they own a pet, the study findings may have underestimated the percentage of respondents who have a significant bond with a companion animal.

Second, the primary variables in the study were measured at the nominal level of measurement. Thus, for example, the findings indicate whether pets were harmed (according to the respondent's understanding of "harm"), but not the number of times an animal was harmed or how seriously the animal was hurt in each incident. Similarly, the findings indicate whether a respondent's concern for pets affected her decision-making, but not the relative importance of concern for pets compared to other factors considered in her decision-making.

Third, the measure of ethnicity was based not on respondents' self-reports but on the observations of staff members who administered the survey. The staff members who recorded the respondents' ethnicity may have relied on language, surname, skin color or other factors to determine a respondent's ethnicity. It is not possible to know whether staff members' designations of ethnicity would match self-reported data. Moreover, as noted in the method section, the staff members who administered the survey failed to record the ethnicity of 11% of the 151 pet owners in the sample.

Data collection. The researchers relied on staff members of the agencies to administer the questionnaires to the clients who agreed to participate. Because of turnover in agency staff, not all staff members who administered the instrument were trained by the researchers. No information was available on the number of women who declined to participate in the survey. Most important, many questionnaires were not fully completed, which resulted in missing data on many survey items.

Implications for Research

Consistent with national data on pet ownership (Pew Research Center, 2006), Hispanic women in the sample were less likely than non-Hispanic women to own pets. Moreover, over half (52.4%) of the non-Hispanic women, compared to a third (32.4%) of the Hispanic women, reported that their partners abused their pets. Although this difference was not statistically significant, potential ethnic differences in batterers' pet abuse warrant additional exploration in samples that adequately represent both Hispanic and non-Hispanic women and include a measure of the perpetrator's ethnicity as well as the female victim's. Such studies should also control for other variables (e.g., income, family size, woman's attachment to pets) to determine whether these factors explain any apparent relationship between ethnicity and partner's pet abuse.

Children's involvement in witnessing and perpetrating pet abuse, as well as their role in protecting family pets, should also be thoroughly explored in future research on IPV in Hispanic families. An important question is whether batterers are *more* or *less* likely to abuse family pets when children are living in the home.

As previously noted, acculturation and immigration status have been associated with vulnerability to IPV among Latinas in the U.S. Are these factors also associated with the co-occurrence of IPV and pet abuse in Hispanic families? What other cultural or social structural factors explain batterers' use of pet abuse as a control strategy in Hispanic families? Finally, research on the meaning of pet ownership and attachment to pets in Hispanic families can contribute to the development of assessment instruments that elicit accurate information about the nature and extent of pet abuse perpetrated by batterers or other family members including children. More accurate assessments enable service providers to help women develop safety plans that include the needs of pets and to develop "safe pet" programs for abused or "at risk" pets. Accurate assessments of children's involvement in pet abuse as witnesses, protectors, or perpetrators can contribute to the development of intervention programs in shelters for children of IPV survivors. In short, research designed to examine the role of pets and the dynamics of pet abuse in Hispanic families can contribute to the development of more culturally competent assessment and intervention services to benefit Hispanic survivors of IPV, their children, and their pets.

AUTHOR NOTE

Catherine A. Faver, PhD, LMSW, is Professor of Social Work at the University of Texas-Pan American. Her research focuses on animal abuse and family violence and on spirituality and social work.

Alonzo M. Cavazos, Jr., EdD, LCSW, is Associate Professor of Social Work at the University of Texas-Pan American. His research focuses on traditional healing among Latinos and on field instruction in social work education.

REFERENCES

Adams, C. J. (1995). Woman-battering and harm to animals. In C. J. Adams & J. Donovan (Eds.), *Animals and women: Feminist theoretical explorations* (pp. 55-84). Durham, NC: Duke University Press.

American Veterinary Medical Association (AVMA). (2002). *U.S. pet ownership & demographics sourcebook.* Schaumburg, IL: Author.

Andersen, M. L., & Collins, P. H. (1998). *Race, class and gender: An anthology.* Belmont, CA: Wadsworth Publishing Co.

Ascione, F. R. (1998). Battered women's reports of their partners and their children's cruelty to animals. *Journal of Emotional Abuse, 1*(1), 199-133.

Ascione, F. R. (2000). *Safe havens for pets: Guidelines for programs sheltering pets for women who are battered.* Logan, UT: Author.

Ascione, F. R. (2005). *Children and animals: Exploring the roots of kindness and cruelty.* West Lafayette, IN: Purdue University Press.

Ascione, F. R., Weber, C. V., & Wood, D. S. (1997, April 25). *Final report on the project: Animal welfare and domestic violence.* Submitted to the Geraldine R. Dodge Foundation. Logan, UT: Authors.

Bachman, R. (1994). *Violence against women: A National Crime Victimization Survey report* (NCJ-145325). Washington, DC: U.S. Department of Justice.

Caetano, R., Schafer, J., Clark, C., Cunradi, C., & Raspberry, K. (2000). Intimate partner violence, acculturation and alcohol consumption among Hispanic couples in the United States. *Journal of Interpersonal Violence, 15*, 30-45.

Falicov, C. (1998). *Latino families in therapy.* New York: Guilford.

Faver, C. A., & Strand, E. B. (2003a). Domestic violence and animal cruelty: Untangling the web of abuse. *Journal of Social Work Education, 39*(2), 237-253.

Faver, C. A., & Strand, E. B. (2003b). To leave or to stay? Battered women's concern for vulnerable pets. *Journal of Interpersonal Violence, 18*(12), 1367-1377.

Faver, C. A., & Strand, E. B. (in press). Unleashing compassion: Social work and animal abuse. In F. R. Ascione (Ed.), *International handbook of theory and research on animal abuse and cruelty.* West Lafayette, IN: Purdue University Press.

Flynn, C. P. (2000a). Battered women and their animal companions: Symbolic interaction between human and nonhuman animals. *Society & Animals, 8*(2), 99-127.

Flynn, C. P. (2000b). Why family professionals can no longer ignore violence toward animals. *Family Relations, 49*(1), 87-95.

Flynn, C. P. (2000c). Woman's best friend: Pet abuse and the role of companion animals in the lives of battered women. *Violence Against Women, 6*(2), 162-177.

Hampton, R. L., & Gelles, R. J. (1994). Violence toward black women in a nationally representative sample of Black families. *Journal of Comparative Family Studies, 25*(1), 105-119.

Humane Society of the United States (HSUS). (2006). *Animal cruelty/domestic violence fact sheet.* Retrieved September 30, 2006, from www.hsus.org/acf/cruelty/publiced.

Johnson, R. A., & Meadows, R. L. (2002). Older Latinos, pets and health. *Western Journal of Nursing Research, 24*, 609-620.

Kantor, G. K., Jasinski, J. L., & Aldarondo, E. (1994). Sociocultural status and incidence of marital violence in Hispanic families. *Violence and Victims, 9*, 207-222.

Kanuha, V. (1994). Women of color in battering relationships. In L. Comas-Diaz & B. Greene (Eds.), *Women of color: Integrating ethnic and gender identities in psychotherapy* (pp. 428-454). New York: Guilford.

Lie, G., & Lowery, C. (2003). Cultural competence with women of color. In D. Lum (Ed.), *Culturally competent practice* (pp. 282-309). Pacific Grove, CA: Brooks/Cole.

Lown, E., & Vega, W. (2001). Prevalence and predictors of physical partner abuse among Mexican American women. *American Journal of Public Health, 91,* 441-446.

McFarlane, J., Parker, B., Koeken, K., & Bullock, L. (1992). Assessing for abuse during pregnancy. *Journal of the American Medical Association, 267,* 3176-3178.

Morash, M., Bui, H. N., & Santiago, A. M. (2000). Cultural-specific gender ideology and wife abuse in Mexican-descent families. *International Review of Victimology, 7,* 67-91.

Neff, J. A., Holamon, B., & Schluter, T. D. (1995). Spousal violence among Anglos, Blacks, and Mexican Americans: The role of demographic variables, psychosocial predictors, and alcohol consumption. *Journal of Family Violence, 19,* 1-25.

Pew Research Center. (2006, March 7). *Gauging family intimacy: Dogs edge cats (dads trail both). A social trends report of the Pew Research Center.* Washington, DC: Pew Research Center.

Quinlisk, J. A. (1999). Animal abuse and family violence. In F. R. Ascione & P. Arkow (Eds.), *Child abuse, domestic violence, and animal abuse* (pp. 168-175). West Lafayette, IN: Purdue University Press.

Ramos, B. M., & Carlson, B. E. (2004). Lifetime abuse and mental health distress among English-speaking Latinas. *Affilia, 19*(3), 239-256.

Rasche, C. E. (2000). Minority women and domestic violence: The unique dilemmas of battered women of color. In H. M. Eigenberg (Ed.), *Women battering in the United States: Till death us do part* (pp. 86-102). Prospect Heights, IL: Waveland Press.

Risley-Curtiss, C., Holley, L. C., Cruickshank, T., Porcelli, J., Rhoads, C., Bacchus, D. N. A. et al. (2006). "She was family": Women of color and animal-human connections. *Affilia: Journal of Women and Social Work,* 21 (4), 433-447.

Risley-Curtiss, C., Holley, L. C., & Wolf, S. (2006). The animal-human bond and ethnic diversity. *Social Work, 51*(3), 257-268.

Siegel, J. M. (1995). Pet ownership and the importance of pets among adolescents. *Anthrozoos, 8*(4), 217-223.

Sorenson, S. B. (1996). Violence against women: Examining ethnic differences and commonalities. *Evaluation Review, 20*(2), 123-145.

Sorenson, S. B., & Telles, C. A. (1991). Self-reports of spousal violence in a Mexican American and non-Hispanic White population. *Violence and Victims, 6,* 3-15.

Sorenson, S. B., Upchurch, D., & Shen, H. (1996). Violence and injury in marital arguments: Risk patterns and gender differences. *American Journal of Public Health, 86,* 35-40.

Strand, E. B. (2003). Battered women's experiences with pet abuse: A survey of women in two domestic violence shelters. *Dissertation Abstracts International, 65*(01A), 290.

Strand, E. B., & Faver, C. A. (2005). Battered women's concern for their pets: A closer look. *Journal of Family Social Work, 9*(4), 39-58.

Straus, M., & Smith, C. (1990). Violence in Hispanic families in the United States: Incidence rates and structural interpretations. In M. A. Straus & R. J. Gelles (Eds.), *Physical violence in American families: Risk factors and adaptations to violence in 8,145 families* (pp. 341-367). New Brunswick, NJ: Transaction.

Texas Council on Family Violence. (2003, May). *Prevalence, perceptions and awareness of domestic violence in Texas: Executive summary.* Retrieved February 16, 2006, from www.tcfv.org.

Texas Council on Family Violence. (2005). *2005 Texas advocates' guide: Family violence laws, policies & protocols.* Austin, TX: Texas Council on Family Violence.

Texas Council on Family Violence. (2006). *Abuse in Texas: 2004 in Texas at a glance.* Retrieved February 16, 2006, from www.tcfv.org/info/abuse_in_texas.html.

Tjaden, P., & Thoennes, N. (1998). *Prevalence, incidence and consequences of violence against women: Findings from the National Violence Against Women Survey.* Denver, CO: Center for Policy Research.

U.S. Census Bureau. (2006). *Quickfacts from the U.S. Census Bureau.* Retrieved February 27, 2006, from www.quickfacts.census.gov/qfd/states.

Vasquez, M. (1994). Latinas. In L. Comas-Diaz & B. Greene (Eds.), *Women of color: Integrating ethnic and gender identities in psychotherapy* (pp. 114-138). New York: Guilford.

West, C., Kantor, G., & Jasinski, J. (1998). Sociodemographic predictors and cultural barriers to help-seeking behavior by Latina and Anglo American battered women. *Violence and Victims, 13*(4), 1-15.

Yllo, K. (1993). Through a feminist lens: Gender, power, and violence. In R. Gelles & D. Loseke (Eds.), *Feminist perspectives on wife abuse* (pp. 28-50). Newbury Park, CA: Sage.

Yoshihama, M. (2000). Reinterpreting strength and safety in a socio-cultural context: Dynamics of domestic violence and experiences of women of Japanese descent. *Children and Youth Services Review, 22*(3/4), 207-229.

doi:10.1300/J135v07n03_04

Child Welfare and Animal Cruelty:
A Survey of Child Welfare Workers

Mary Montminy-Danna

SUMMARY. Twenty-two percent of the child welfare workers surveyed indicated they have been assigned child maltreatment cases where there is a subsequent disclosure of animal cruelty. Both quantitative and qualitative methods were used to understand how the issue of animal cruelty is addressed within the child welfare system. At present there is no standard protocol for inquiring about and addressing the issue of animal cruelty. Some workers have expanded their assessment protocol to include questions about experiences with animal cruelty. Perpetrators include boys, girls, relatives, and caregivers. Challenges for the child welfare system on all system levels are addressed. doi:10.1300/J135v07n03_05 *[Article copies available for a fee from The Haworth Document Delivery Service: 1-800-HAWORTH. E-mail address: <docdelivery@haworthpress.com> Website: <http://www.HaworthPress.com> © 2007 by The Haworth Press. All rights reserved.]*

KEYWORDS. Child welfare, child welfare workers, animal cruelty, LINKS

Address correspondence to: Mary Montminy-Danna, LICSW, PhD (E-mail: montminm@salve.edu).

[Haworth co-indexing entry note]: "Child Welfare and Animal Cruelty: A Survey of Child Welfare Workers." Montminy-Danna, Mary. Co-published simultaneously in *Journal of Emotional Abuse* (The Haworth Maltreatment & Trauma Press, an imprint of The Haworth Press) Vol. 7, No. 3, 2007, pp. 83-96; and: *Animal Abuse and Family Violence: Linkages, Research, and Implications for Professional Practice* (ed: Marti T. Loring, Robert Geffner, and Janessa Marsh) The Haworth Maltreatment & Trauma Press, an imprint of The Haworth Press, 2007, pp. 83-96. Single or multiple copies of this article are available for a fee from The Haworth Document Delivery Service [1-800-HAWORTH, 9:00 a.m. - 5:00 p.m. (EST). E-mail address: docdelivery@haworthpress.com].

INTRODUCTION

It is becoming more widely recognized that there exists a relationship between animal cruelty and family violence (Humane Society of the United States, 2002; Jorgenson & Maloney, 1999). Animal cruelty is found to exist in families where spouses are battered and children are emotionally, physically, and sexually abused (Ascione, 2001; Ascione & Lockwood, 1998; Ascione & Arkow, 1999; Faver & Strand, 2003; Flynn, 2000; Flynn, 1999). Some providers of services to battered women and their children have discovered through research that a number of their residents have had the experience of animal cruelty; sometimes the perpetrator is a child. Both females and males have been found to abuse animals; however, boys are more often offenders than are girls (Humane Society of the United States, 2002, 2003, 2004; Jorgenson & Maloney, 1999). Other times, the population of non-sheltered abused mothers will recount episodes of animal cruelty that have occurred in their homes while their children observed. When prompted in a safe environment, children of battered women were found to recount their experiences with animal cruelty (Montminy-Danna & Rice, 1999).

A number of mental health workers and law enforcement officials now recognize and acknowledge the link among various forms of interpersonal and companion animal violence. Frequently, animal control officers are involved in removing a companion pet from a house where there is evidence of child maltreatment. During this process, it sometimes comes to the attention of the animal control officer that the children living in the household may also be in need of services (Arkow, 1995, 2002).

Partnerships between animal welfare organizations and child welfare organizations are beginning to evolve and examine the connection and overlap of cases (Zilney & Zilney, 2005; Becker & French, 2004; Zilney & Ronald, 2002). Trainings designed for social service providers, animal control officers, and veterinarians exploring the connections are beginning to be made available in a few communities, and models for addressing the issue of animal cruelty have been developed (personal communication, Barbara Walsh, 2005). Some emphasize the need to educate future human service professionals on this issue (Faver & Strand, 2005; Becker & French, 2004). Child welfare workers are beginning to recognize that where there is violence towards children, there is sometimes the concern for the family pets. Zilney and Zilney (2005), in their study of cross-reporting between child welfare workers and humane services workers, found that the child welfare workers noted concerns for the family animals in 20% of cases. An enormous challenge facing child welfare organizations charged with providing substitutive care for children is especially daunting when the children or their families have a history of hurting or killing animals. Placing children with such a history in a group home, relative care, or foster care may very well put both the humans and animals at risk.

Overview of the Problem: The Continuum of Violence and Perpetrator

The impact on children as victims and perpetrators of animal cruelty is an area within the social service that deserves more attention. Specifically, there is a lack of evidence showing the direct biological, emotional, and social consequences for children associated with animal cruelty. It is widely believed that children living with trauma will be negatively affected in one or more domains of their lives. This study and numerous others have looked at the issue of animal cruelty in the context of multiple forms of family violence.

Children living with or who have experienced family violence are at risk for becoming victims, abusers, and sometimes both. Children may attempt to cope with their own victimization through a variety of means (Joseph, Govender, & Bhagwanjee, 2006). Children have been found to be more aggressive towards animals if they have been exposed to violence within the home (Currie, 2006). Victims of exposure to violence or assault frequently exhibit symptoms of living with trauma and have been found to show signs of aggression, use drugs and/or alcohol, and are more often truant (Montminy-Danna, 1997). Others show poor concentration, lowered verbal functioning, and less than adequate school performance (Ybarra, Wilkens & Lieberman, 2006; Montminy-Danna, 1997). Children may also turn inward with feelings of depression and withdrawal and may experience thoughts of suicide or display suicidal gestures. The symptoms may be protracted and last well beyond the course of exposure to violence. Therefore, removal from the traumatic situation doesn't necessarily result in a slowing down or arresting of symptoms.

For those that are perpetrators of violence, many have violent histories. Beginning in the 1970s, the FBI began to compile profiles of serial killers and noted that a common feature of all cases was that there had been a history of animal cruelty. Since then a number of more recent cases, such as those involving school shooters, have again shown where notorious killers had a past that included instances of violence towards animals (Arkow, 2002; Merz-Perez, Heide, Silverman, 2001). We've only recently understood that this past aggression towards animals could be an indicator of serious harm to humans.

Measuring Animal Cruelty

It is very hard to accurately measure episodes of animal cruelty because of the nature of the problem. Sometimes the harming or killing of animals is not regarded as a problem behavior or an act of cruelty. Animal cruelty is often minimized or seen as something "children, especially boys, just do." Even when it is recognized, parents, guardians, social service workers, or law enforcement don't necessarily attend to the problem after the first assault. Nor in the case of child welfare does it necessarily come to the attention of case workers during the intake and assessment process. Rather, information about a child's experience as a witness or perpetrator of animal cruelty is discovered largely by chance. These revelations might be in the form of self or parent report, discovered by a worker with insight about the prevalence, or perhaps because a report to the social service agency has been made with regard to a child in their care. However, opportunities for gathering this information are beginning to surface, and we are beginning to have a fuller understanding of the needs of children. In dealing with mothers of children exposed to domestic violence, it was found that mothers are more likely to disclose incidents of animal cruelty when they have a chance to both develop a rapport with workers and when they understand the range of acts relative to animal cruelty (Montminy-Danna & Rice, 1999).

The focus of this research was to answer the following question: *What is the prevalence of animal cruelty in the cases of families served by the state child welfare organization?* Subsequent questions that the study attempted to answer included identifying the perpetrator of animal cruelty and gaining insight as to how the presence of animal cruelty affects placement decisions. Lastly, a driving force behind this inquiry was to learn more about the needs of families involved in the state child welfare organization and how the state child welfare organization can better address those needs.

METHODS

A brief five-question survey (Initial Caseworker Survey) was distributed to family service workers, intake workers, and juvenile probation officers employed by the state child welfare organization. Since there is not a specific question regarding animal cruelty asked by the child welfare department, the sample was chosen based on the understanding that any of these individuals, in their role with the department as a direct service worker, may have acquired anecdotal information about animal cruelty. The survey inquired about cases involving animal cruelty for the previous calendar year. A cover letter was sent along with the survey describing the research. At first, the cover letter and survey were emailed. As a follow-up, reminder emails were sent and to increase participation, hard copies of the survey were distributed to each field office in the four regions making up the statewide organization. Specifically, the questions asked about cases involving animal cruelty, the percentage of cases, protocol for documenting animal cruelty and interest in participating in follow-up interviews (see Table 1).

Follow-up interviews and focus groups were held with a sample of those individuals who completed the survey. Participants were invited based on their responses to the initial survey, which asked if they would be willing to provide more detailed information about their experiences with cases involving animal cruelty. Because of the brevity of the survey, follow-ups were convened to further understand the breadth and depth of the experiences of the individual workers. Two focus groups (comprised of four child welfare workers, a training specialist, and the interviewer) and four individual interviews were held. The individuals represented the diversity of the population served. Some noted that they worked with families in an urban setting, others in a suburban setting, and still others worked with families living in rural parts of the state. A set of questions was used to facilitate the group and individual discussions. The questions addressed the ways in which animal cruelty is identified, the time and manner which disclosure occurs, co-existing issues, types of animals and injuries, information about the perpetrator, and implications for practice (see Table 2).

FINDINGS

Quantitative Findings

Family service workers, intake workers, juvenile probation officers, and counselors from the juvenile secure detention facility ($N = 500$) were sent email surveys and then follow-up hard copies of the survey during the summer and fall of 2002. A total of 121 surveys were re-

TABLE 1. Initial Caseworker Survey

1. Are you aware of incidences of animal cruelty in your caseload during the last calendar
   year 2001-2002?

2. What percentage of your caseload do you estimate had issues related to animal cruelty
   during the calendar year 2001-2002?

3. Did you document information related to animal cruelty in your case during the calendar
   year 2001-2002?

4. If you answered Yes to Question 3, where did you document this information in the case
   record (i.e., Case Activity Notes, Case Profile Narrative, etc.)?

5. If you answered Yes to Question 1, would you be willing to give us more details about
   these cases?

turned. Of those, 111 were used in the research analyses (10 were found to be duplicates and therefore dropped from the analysis). Of those reporting their gender, 14 were male and 84 were female. Twenty-two and one-half percent of the respondents indicated that they had cases involving animal cruelty during the previous year (see Figure 1). The majority of the returns (> 95%) came from the family service workers who represent the majority of workers within the child welfare system. Of those, three respondents indicated that between 1-2% of cases involved animal cruelty, 18 indicated that between 5-12% of their cases involved animal cruelty, and four individuals said that 13-25% of their caseload involved animal cruelty (see Figure 2). All but three of the respondents indicated that they documented the animal cruelty somewhere in the client file. Most recorded the information in the case activity file and in at least one other location.

Qualitative Interviews

Two focus groups were held with individuals representing one-half of the statewide reporting regions. Additionally, extensive phone interviews were held with individuals who were unable to attend the focus groups but had indicated that some of their cases involved animal cruelty. All individuals involved in the interviews were female. The fol-

TABLE 2. Follow-Up Caseworker Questionnaire

1. How do issues of animal cruelty get raised within the context of cases?

2. In general, how does the animal cruelty change the nature of your practice? What, if any, challenges are raised with this issue?

3. Does the time at which the disclosure occurs make a difference?

4. Who is identified as the perpetrator of the animal cruelty?

5. Are there factors that co-exist with the issues of animal cruelty? If so, what are they?

6. Did the child witness cruelty to the family pets by a caregiver?

7. What form of cruelty occurred (threat, harm/injury, death)?

8. Please describe the specifics.

9. How many pets have been threatened, injured or harmed?

10. Was a report made to an animal control officer?

11. What was the age of the child when the animal cruelty occurred?

12. Was there any disclosure of domestic violence?

13. If so, was the child a witness to the domestic violence?

14. Are there barriers to case management because of the existence of animal cruelty?

15. What recommendations do you have for the researcher/child welfare department with respect to cases involving animal cruelty?

lowing is a summary of the information gathered during both the individual and group sessions. All of the individuals in attendance had at least one case that involved animal cruelty. Many had encountered numerous cases throughout their careers. In addition to questions posed by the researcher, the focus group participants provided information relative to the specifics of their cases, procedures employed when information about animal cruelty is disclosed, the impact on their practice, and suggestions for future practice.

Entry into child welfare services. Cases do not come to the attention of child welfare because of animal cruelty. Rather, disclosures about an-

FIGURE 1. Child Welfare Workers' Reports of Animal Cruelty

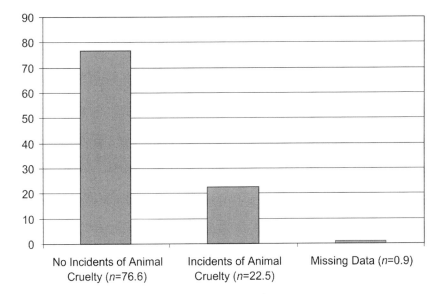

imal cruelty generally occur after the family has become involved with the child welfare department. Disclosures have come from a child, parent, sibling or foster family. Other times a worker has questioned a family member about current or past family pets or the observation of a pet has led a worker to pursue information about the health and well being of the pet(s).

Documenting animal abuse. At present there is no statutory or regulatory mandate for reporting animal abusers. Therefore, inquiry about animal abuse is not required. There is not a specific question on the intake form; however, the opportunity to document information about animal cruelty can be documented if a worker chooses to do so. Workers indicated that they did document the cruelty of pets or death of pets. It was documented in either the case narrative or social history sections of the family file.

Types of abuse. A distinction was made between animals in the home and animals in the community. The reports captured a range of varied incidents from neglect to deliberate physical abuse and sexual abuse of the animal. Withholding food, exercise, and water was a common finding. Rough handling of all types of animals occurred; this includes throwing the animal and pulling ears, tails, and fur. Dogs were burned

FIGURE 2. Percentage of Child Welfare Workers' Caseload Including Animal Cruelty (*n* = 25)

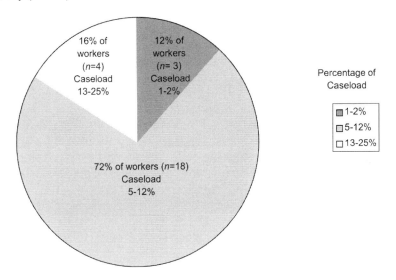

and stomped on. Cats were drowned and slammed on the ground. The necks of cats, rabbits, and birds were snapped, resulting in death of the animal. In some instances, children were observed sexually molesting the dog or cat.

Children and adolescents were found to also hurt animals in the wild. Animals such as frogs, squirrels, rabbits, and waterfowl were captured and killed. Some of the children attempted to hide the remains of the animals in the home while others openly displayed the carnage. The availability of animals seemed to play a role in whether acts were committed on domestic (pets) or animals in the community or in the wild.

Perpetrators of cruelty. This study found that cases had identified various persons as the perpetrator. In some instances the perpetrator was a child; other times it was an adult caregiver (parent, grandparent, adult sibling). Sometimes it was done in a discreet manner, while other times pets were harmed in the presence of others, including workers. Children of all ages have been identified as abusers (Humane Society of the United States, 2002, 2003, 2004; Jorgenson & Maloney, 1999). In this study the range of ages was from 3 to 18. An equal number of females and males were identified as abusers.

Emotional and psychological consequences. The harming or killing of pets is used as a mechanism to ensure that children will submit to certain behaviors or be made to keep secrets. Caregivers were found hurt, threaten, or kill a pet in the presence of a child to ensure that the child was scared into silence or compliance. Most of the cases in this study involved physical and/or sexual abuse of the child or children (Ascione & Lockwood, 1998; Ascione & Arkow, 1999; Faver & Strand, 2003; Flynn, 2000). Caregivers used the threat of the harm or killing of the animal to ensure that the child would not disclose the sexual abuse that was happening to them. In fact, all interviewees stated that a disclosure of animal cruelty was considered a red flag that prompted the worker to take a closer look as to whether the child (in care of the child welfare department for neglect or physical abuse) might also be a victim of sexual abuse.

The endless cycle of pets. The child welfare workers found that many of the families with whom they worked had a history of owning multiple pets. Some workers found that when such a history was taken, families often had numerous pets at the time, replaced pets over and over again, and in some instances indicated that the pets had disappeared, run away, or had died.

Impact on practice. All child welfare workers agreed that cases involving both child maltreatment and animal cruelty were some of the most challenging to deal with. Some workers have developed their own best practices for intervening with cases involving animal cruelty. Some reported removing the animals to alternative settings that would provide appropriate care. These settings included shelters, the homes of workers, or animal loving friends. When the child is being removed to a foster home or in foster care when the disclosure is made, consideration about the potential for harm to the foster family's pet(s) becomes a central issue for the worker. All of the workers who knew there was a history of animal cruelty said that they discussed this matter with the foster home and would address the matter directly with the child. When there was knowledge of animal cruelty, careful supervision of the child when around the family pet was also recommended. Others became aware of the animal cruelty after a child was in foster care. In most of these cases, it was an incident by the child toward the foster pet that brought the problem to light.

Recommendations by workers. Many workers suggested that mandatory training on animal cruelty be provided to the current staff and to new workers. The training should include an overview of the issues of animal cruelty, the connection to family violence, and methods of assessment and treatment. Others reported that they were unaware of existing resources that address the complex needs of animals and families and needed information in that regard. Still others suggested the establishment of groups for animal abusers, especially when the perpetrator is a minor. Some mentioned that the initial contact by the Child Protective Investigator should include an inquiry about pets in the home. Others suggested adding a question to the intake form that not only asked about the current pets but also behaviors toward past pets and animals.

DISCUSSION

These findings present a number of challenges to child welfare organizations and highlight the need for further research in this area. The response rate was under 25% and therefore is limited in its ability to be generalized. Secondly, it is possible that "animal cruelty" might be a relatively new concept and therefore not universally understood. In the future, a more comprehensive definition should be provided to those surveyed. This study found that a large number of the child welfare cases involve animal cruelty (Human Society of the United States, 2002; Jorgenson & Maloney, 1999). Over 22% of child welfare workers responding to the survey reported having cases that included animal cruelty. Because of the high incidence of child welfare cases involving animal cruelty, it is important that training on the connections or links be provided to all workers involved at every stage of child welfare delivery. Workers need assistance in the recognition, assessment, and intervention of animal cruelty (Faver & Strand, 2003).

Earlier detection would assist in better treatment planning and intervention. Some workers spoke of the problems created for foster families with pets in the home when a disclosure was made subsequent to the placement of a child. Some of these situations would be better managed by having upfront knowledge. Questions about animal cruelty should be included on current intake forms and should be asked early on in the helping process. This will systematically apprise the workers, potential placements, and counselors of important information needed to support children and families in the child welfare system. Workers who have encountered incidents of animal cruelty in prior cases are likely to inquire about the issue in each case they are assigned.

This study shows that the perpetrator is just as likely to be a female as a male. Reports of girls and female caregivers as the offender raise questions about the typical animal abuser profile. This finding also brings into question a potential bias that may exist within child welfare, one that underestimates the behavior of young girls in this regard. This has implications for work with families from the aspect of inquiry to creating gender-appropriate interventions.

Work within the child welfare system to address the needs of animal-abusing individuals requires linkages outside of the system. It is imperative that animal shelters, domestic violence treatment providers, law enforcement, veterinarians, and the mental health community unite in an effort to share resources and develop policy initiatives that promote safe families.

CONCLUSIONS

This study highlights the needs of workers at the individual and agency level and informs practice that will address the unique needs of families with a history of animal cruelty. The present climate seems to be one in which child welfare workers are beginning to acknowledge and attempting to address issues of animal cruelty as it relates to their casework with children and families. The complex nature of animal cruelty, coupled with the presence of child maltreatment, necessitates an approach that is comprehensive and may involve linking with resources outside of the child welfare domain. Developing partnerships with other agencies providing protection to humans and animals is essential for developing a best practice approach.

AUTHOR NOTE

Mary Montminy-Danna, LICSW, PhD, is Assistant Professor of Social Work at Salve Regina University in Newport, Rhode Island. She has held that appointment for the past 18 years. Her major responsibilities include teaching practice and policy courses and coordinating the field experience for junior and senior social work majors. She is currently the clinical consultant for the Women's Resource Center of Newport and Bristol Counties, Inc. Ms. Montminy-Danna is a trainer for the State of Rhode Island on the LINKS between animal cruelty and interpersonal violence. She has conducted research in this area and on children living with violence and school performance.

REFERENCES

Arkow, P. (1995). *Breaking the cycles of violence: A practical guide.* Alameda, CA: The Latham Foundation.
Arkow, P. (2002). *Breaking the cycles of violence: A guide to multi-disciplinary interventions.* Alameda, CA: The Latham Foundation.

Ascione, F. R. (2001). Animal abuse and youth violence. *Juvenile Justice Bulletin.*

Ascione, F. R., & Arkow, P. (Eds.). (1999). *Child abuse, domestic violence and animal abuse: Linking the circles of compassion for prevention and intervention.* West Lafayette, IN: Purdue University Press.

Ascione, F. R., & Lockwood, R. (Eds.). (1998). *Cruelty to animals and interpersonal violence: Readings in research and application.* West Lafayette, IN: Purdue University Press.

Becker, F., & French, L. (2004). Child abuse, animal cruelty and domestic violence. *Child Abuse Review, 13*(6), 399-414.

Currie, C. (2006). Animal cruelty by children exposed to family violence. *Child Abuse and Neglect, 30*(4), 425-435.

Faver, C. A., & Strand, E. L. (2003). Domestic violence and animal cruelty: Untangling the web of violence. *Journal of Social Work Education, 39*(2), 237-254.

Flynn, C. P. (1999). Exploring the link between corporal punishment and children's cruelty to animals. *Journal of Marriage and Family, 61*(4), 971-981.

Flynn, C. P. (2000). Why family professionals can no longer ignore violence toward animals. *Family Relations, 49*(1), 87-95.

Humane Society of the United States. (2002). *First Strike Champagne 2001 report of animal cruelty cases.* Washington, DC: Author.

Humane Society of the United States. (2003). *First Strike Champagne 2002 report of animal cruelty cases.* Washington, DC: Author.

Humane Society of the United States. (2004). *First Strike Champagne 2003 report of animal cruelty cases.* Washington, DC: Author.

Jorgenson, S., & Maloney, L. (1999). Animal abuse and the victims of domestic violence. In F. R. Ascione & P. Arkow (Eds.), *Child abuse, domestic violence, and animal abuse* (pp. 143-158). West Lafayette, IN: Purdue University Press.

Joseph, S., Govender, K., & Bhagwanjee, A. (2006). "I can't see him hit her again, I just want to run away . . . hide and block my ears": A phenomenological analysis of a sample of children's coping responses to exposure to domestic violence. *Journal of Emotional Abuse, 6*(4), 23-45.

Merz-Perez, L., Heide, K. M., & Silverman, I. J. (2001). Childhood cruelty to animals and subsequent violence against humans. *International Journal of Offender Therapy and Comparative Criminology, 45*(5), 556-573.

Montminy-Danna, M. L. (1997). *Evaluation report: A comparative study of school performance of children who witness family violence and their non-reporting agemates.* Conducted for the Mental Health Association of Rhode Island.

Montminy-Danna, M. L., & Rice, H. (1999). Children with domestic violence and animal cruelty. Published in the *International Conference on Children Exposed to Domestic Violence Conference Proceedings.* B.C./Yukon Society of Transition Houses, Vancouver, B.C.

Walsh, B. (2005). Coordinator of Employee Training, Rhode Island Department of Administration, Office of Training and Development. Personal communication.

Ybarra, G., Wilkens, S., & Lieberman, A. (2007). The influence of domestic violence on preschooler behavior and functioning. *Journal of Family Violence, 22*(1), 33-42.

Zilney, M., & Ronald, L. (2002, Summer). Examining the link between child and animal welfare in Wellington County, Ontario. *The Latham Letter, XXIII*(3).
Zilney, L. A., & Zilney, M. (2005). Reunification of child welfare and animal welfare
   agencies: Cross-reporting of abuse in Wellington County, Ontario. *Child Welfare,
   84*(1), 47-66.

doi:10.1300/J135v07n03_05

Integrating Animals
into the Family Violence Paradigm:
Implications for Policy
and Professional Standards

Mary Lou Randour

SUMMARY. Noting the established link between animal abuse and family violence, this paper outlines the implications for policy and professional standards. Federal policies related to the collection of crime statistics by the Federal Bureau of Investigation, as well as the collection by federal agencies of data on family violence, including domestic abuse and child abuse and neglect, are cited and proposals for including questions about animal cruelty into these federal databases are offered. Various types of state legislation, such as cross reporting and increased penalties for individuals who commit violence in the presence of minors, are described, and the implications for the link between animal abuse and family violence are discussed. Finally, the important area of professional standards–how the mental health profession sets and maintains standards for education and training–is reviewed and suggestions for

Address correspondence to: Mary Lou Randour, PhD (E-mail: Randour@comcast.net).

[Haworth co-indexing entry note]: "Integrating Animals into the Family Violence Paradigm: Implications for Policy and Professional Standards." Randour, Mary Lou. Co-published simultaneously in *Journal of Emotional Abuse* (The Haworth Maltreatment & Trauma Press, an imprint of The Haworth Press) Vol. 7, No. 3, 2007, pp. 97-116; and: *Animal Abuse and Family Violence: Linkages, Research, and Implications for Professional Practice* (ed: Marti T. Loring, Robert Geffner, and Janessa Marsh) The Haworth Maltreatment & Trauma Press, an imprint of The Haworth Press, 2007, pp. 97-116. Single or multiple copies of this article are available for a fee from The Haworth Document Delivery Service [1-800-HAWORTH, 9:00 a.m. - 5:00 p.m. (EST). E-mail address: docdelivery@haworthpress.com].

the inclusion of animal cruelty as an important component for assessment and treatment are proposed. doi:10.1300/J135v07n03_06 *[Article copies available for a fee from The Haworth Document Delivery Service: 1-800-HAWORTH. E-mail address: <docdelivery@haworthpress.com> Website: <http://www.HaworthPress.com> © 2007 by The Haworth Press. All rights reserved.]*

KEYWORDS. Animal cruelty, family violence, domestic violence, child abuse, human-animal interaction

John Jefferson pleaded guilty in a Brooklyn courthouse to robbery, burglary, stalking, criminal contempt, and animal cruelty. Jefferson, who had been stalking his ex-girlfriend Eugenia Miller, had hurled Ribsy, a 16-year-old terrier poodle mix of Miller's, off her balcony. State Supreme Court Justice James Yates sentenced Jefferson to 12 years in prison; the judge said that two were for Rigby.

The case of John Jefferson dramatically illustrates two points: the close connection between animal abuse and family violence and how the enforcement of animal cruelty laws can not only protect animals, but also families. Other authors in this issue offer detailed information on the link between animal abuse and family violence (see Schaefer, Onyskiw, this volume). The link between animal abuse and domestic violence, a topic that has attracted numerous research studies, has been firmly established over the last 20 years: "(P)et abuse is common in the lives of significant proportions of battered women and in a number of cases (18-48%) concern for pets' welfare affected women's decisions about whether to enter or the timing of entry into domestic violence shelters" (Ascione et al., 2007, p. 3). Previous studies on the connection between animal abuse and domestic violence, as Ascione noted in his most recent study (2007), have been limited by their reliance on anecdotal reports, use of convenience samples, and small samples sizes. Two recent studies, however, have overcome the limitations of the earlier studies, thereby providing firmer evidence of the association of intimate partner violence (IPV) with animal abuse. Comparing a group of women residing in domestic violence shelters, Ascione and his colleagues found that these women were nearly 11 times more likely to report that their partner had hurt or killed pets than a comparison group of women who had not experienced intimate partner violence (Ascione et al., 2007).

The significance of pet abuse to family violence also was confirmed by a recent gold standard study that sought to identify risk factors for partners perpetrating IPV. The case-control study of 3,627 women and 845 controls was conducted from 1994 to 2000 in 11 United States metropolitan cities (Walton-Moss, Manganello, Frye, & Campbell, 2005). Pet abuse was one of four risk factors identified for IPV. In addition to the identification of pet abuse, the other three factors included not being a high school graduate, being in fair or poor mental health, and having a problem with drug or alcohol use.

Although the link between animal abuse and child abuse has gained acceptance in the research and practice communities, it is interesting to note that there are very few studies published in scholarly journals that demonstrate such a link. The most frequently cited study on this topic was one conducted in 1983 of 53 families under investigation for suspected child abuse (DeViney, Dickert, & Lockwood, 1983). The investigators found that pet abuse was documented in 60% of the families surveyed and in 88% of those families under supervision for physical abuse.

Despite the lack of empirical documentation of this link, there are other means to make the judgment that an important link does exist between child abuse and animal abuse. In 1998, Howard Davidson, Center for Children and the Law, American Bar Association, wrote an article about the link between animal cruelty and child maltreatment. In it he noted that although animal abuse is an underreported problem, animal cruelty has been used in criminal prosecutions. In one case, a court joined two charges, one for child neglect and the other for animal mistreatment, at one trial as if they were the same act or transaction. A threat of animal abuse to silence child sex abuse victims also has been a factor in a number of criminal convictions (Davidson, 1998).

Also, by way of analogy, the research linking intimate partner violence (IPV) with child maltreatment makes the case that animal abuse is a family matter. By using samples derived from child welfare systems to identify the incidence of IPV, and the use of domestic violence and homeless shelter samples to document the occurrence of child maltreatment, one often-cited study found that domestic violence and child maltreatment overlaps in between 30 to 60 percent of families (Edelson, 1999).

As Renner and Slack (2004) note, the two systems of domestic violence and child maltreatment do not collect data on violence that is undetected by the other system. As a consequence, "these rates probably overstate the *rate* of co-occurrence in a more general population, (however) they clearly underestimate the *number* of cases in which both forms of violence occur" (p. 2).

Still another signal that practitioners recognize the reality that animals are a part of the family violence equation has been the development of "Safe Haven" programs. These programs provide for sheltering of the pets of domestic violence victims, typically through a cooperative effort between a domestic violence agency and animal sheltering organization. The existence of these programs, and their rapid expansion across the country, reflect the growing awareness of the role of pets in the dynamic of family violence and provide a practical solution to one aspect of this problem: allowing women to feel free to leave a dangerous situation without fear for their pets' safety (Ascione, 2000).

Concomitant with the greater recognition of interpersonal violence as a serious societal problem has been the increased awareness of the importance of examining *all* forms of family violence (Renner & Slack, 2004). There is growing agreement that approaches to domestic violence, child and elder abuse and neglect need to examine violence in the larger context of families for purposes of identification, treatment, or legal responses, rather than to treat the types of violence as distinct, non-overlapping categories. Attention is being directed at the necessity to develop and implement interventions from an "ecological framework," i.e., based on the individual, family and community (McKinney, Sieger, Agliata, & Renk, 2005).

Despite this progress in the conceptualization and response to family and youth violence, there is still a persistent lack of systematic attention being paid to one important category of family and community violence–animal cruelty–and the integral role that animal cruelty crimes plays in the prevention and treatment of violence. The following section will offer detailed examples of how policy and practice can integrate animal cruelty into approaches to family violence.

IMPLICATIONS FOR POLICY, LEGISLATION, AND PROFESSIONAL STANDARDS

As noted earlier, research clearly demonstrates (and common sense dictates) that children who witness violence in the family are at greater risk. One way in which children too frequently witness violence in families, and are subjected to a form of indirect violence themselves, occurs when children observe animal abuse. In the recent study noted earlier (Ascione et al., 2007), 61.54% of the children of domestic violence victims witnessed pet abuse compared to 2.9% of children in the control group. Shelter-group children were more likely to exhibit problem behavior and to have a history of abusing animals themselves.

To successfully integrate animals into the research, policy, and practice of the family violence field will require changes at many levels: federal, state, and professional. The following discussion proposes specific ways in which federal and state actions, as well as changes in professional standards, could advance this integration of animals into the thinking about, and approaches to, family violence. Moreover, the discussion details how such an integration of animal welfare into human welfare responses would strengthen protection and enhance interventions for all members of society.

Federal Policies

Increasingly, policy makers and practitioners are recognizing that the crime and behavior of animal cruelty, and its many implications for child development, juvenile delinquency, and family violence, and other crime, is a significant problem that needs to be addressed. For example, 42 states and the District of Columbia now have felony provisions in their animal cruelty laws. Felony provisions encourage the investigation and prosecution of animal cruelty cases.

Since animal cruelty is so often linked to other types of crime (e.g., family violence, drug and substance abuse violence toward others, and offenses against property [Arluke & Luke, 1997]), these strengthened animal cruelty laws offer police agencies and prosecutor's offices more tools with which to investigate and try cases. Although these felony animal cruelty laws are an important addition, their effectiveness has been mitigated by the failure of juvenile and adult crime data reporting systems to establish a separate category of crime for animal cruelty. This failure has many serious implications for law enforcement as well as the animal and human service communities.

Once a problem, like animal cruelty, has been identified, it is necessary that researchers, policy makers, and practitioners be able to gather data about it, track it, and plan effective interventions. Although local police departments document animal cruelty arrests and convictions for both juveniles and adults, they do not have a crime data collection system into which animal cruelty crimes can be entered as a discrete category. For example, in Montgomery County, Maryland, the police department (MCPD) enters animal cruelty crimes under the category, "Other traffic offenses," making it impossible to disaggregate data on animal cruelty offenses once collected.

Data collection for animal cruelty crimes. The Federal Bureau of Investigation (FBI) determines what crimes are tracked and the definitions for identified crimes. These crime categories and definitions, in turn, are used by state law enforcement agencies to report their crime data to the FBI. The FBI's crime data reporting program is a nationwide effort that collects crime statistics from nearly 17,000 local and state law enforcement agencies. In 2000, the participating agencies represented 94 percent of the U.S. population (Office of Juvenile Justice and Delinquency Prevention, 2006).

Reported crimes vary from criminal homicide in Part I to curfew and loitering laws in Part II. Law enforcement, criminologists, legislators, sociologists, municipal planners, the media, and others interested in criminal justice use the statistics for research and planning purposes. However, under the current FBI crime data reporting system, there is no category to report crimes of animal cruelty. Although crimes of animal cruelty, some of them felonies, are being recorded by local and state police agencies, they have no category established by the FBI in which to place them. In the example cited earlier of the Montgomery County Police Department in Maryland, there have been several successful prosecutions using felony-level animal cruelty laws adopted by Maryland in 2002, yet this data will be absorbed into information about traffic offenses.

Without such knowledge, responders are operating in the dark, without the necessary knowledge they would need to plan effective prevention and intervention strategies. In the last 20 years, we have witnessed a vigorous response to youth violence and domestic violence. Alarmed by the rapid increase in youth violence in the 1980s, federal resources were directed at developing a better understanding of the causes of the problem and the identification of effective interventions for it. As a result, 2003 witnessed the ninth consecutive year of decline in the Violent Crime Index. Between 1994 and 2003, the juvenile arrest rate for Violent Crime Index fell 48%, its lowest level since 1980 (Snyder, 2005).

Devoting resources to a problem helps. One result of this concentrated attention to the problem of youth violence was the development of Blueprints for Violence Prevention Initiative, launched in 1996 by The Center for the Study and Prevention of Violence (CSPV). After conducting a national review, 11 youth violence prevention and intervention programs that met a rigorous scientific standard for program effectiveness were chosen. The 11 model programs, or Blueprints, have been proven to be effective in reducing violent adolescent crime (Center for the Study and Prevention of Violence, 2006). Similar trends can be found in family violence. The rate of family violence fell between 1993 and 2002 from an estimated 5.4 victims to 2.1 victims per 1,000 U. S. residents age 12 or older (Durose et al., 2005).

The advances made in addressing youth and family violence confirm the assertion that "access to sound data is an integral aspect of assessing and addressing any problem effectively" (Flores, 2003). The omission of animal cruelty statistics from the FBI crime data reporting system, however, prevents access to "sound data" and therefore to the vital information needed to design, implement, and evaluate interventions.

Assigning the crime of animal cruelty to its own classification would have a number of advantages. Law enforcement agencies, researchers, policy planners, and others would be better able to understand the factors associated with animal abuse, track trends at the state and national level, and determine the demographic characteristics associated with animal abuse, all of which would assist in promoting more effective intervention and prevention strategies for interrupting the cycle of violence.

Officials at the FBI have acknowledged that designating a separate category for animal cruelty crimes in the national indices initiative now being developed would add considerably more data analysis capabilities: ". . . variables such as felony animal abuse arrests could be linked with a vast array of other statistics to develop useful demographic information" (Letter from Michael D. Kirkpatrick, FBI, to U. S. Senator Paul Sarbanes, September 30, 2003). The expanded databases of the new system would enable law enforcement agencies to identify and track individuals with histories of violence.

Following the lead of the FBI, state law enforcement agencies do not collect or report animal cruelty crimes when collecting and analyzing juvenile crime statistics. The Office of Juvenile Justice and Delinquency Prevention (OJJDP) compiles arrest information and traces the trends, rates, and statistics of juvenile criminal activity. Crime categories include crimes of violence, property offenses, and Status Offenses (e.g., truancy, curfew violations). A social policy programmer who wanted information for planning an anti-youth violence campaign could determine how much vagrancy, vandalism, and suspicious behaviors occurred among adolescents in an identified area. However, since animal cruelty crimes are recorded in the category of "all other offenses" and does not have its own separate category, it is not possible to analyze data on animal cruelty offenses, even though they are linked to many other crimes and are an early indicator of an at-risk child.

There is now scientific consensus that earlier interventions with children and families are more effective and that the development of disruptive and delinquent behavior takes place in a progressive fashion (Kelley, Loeber, Keenan, & DeLamatre, 1997). Animal cruelty often is one of the first indicators of a disruption in development or a problem in the family. A recent analysis of a 20-year longitudinal study on the causes and correlates of youth violence determined that animal cruelty was one of four factors associated with the persistence of aggressive and criminal behavior (Loeber, 2004).

Domestic violence data collection. Similarly, the close association of animal abuse with domestic violence has been firmly established, most notably in the two recent studies cited earlier. However, the federal standards for the collection of data on domestic violence fail to mention animal cruelty as a factor to consider. The Centers for Disease Control (CDC) develops and publishes a guidebook for researchers, *Intimate Partner Violence Surveillance: Uniform Definitions and Recommended Data Elements.* This set of recommendations is designed to promote consistency in the use of terminology and data collection related to IPV. Under the CDC framework, violence is divided into four abuse categories: physical, sexual, threat of physical or sexual, and psychological/emotional (Saltzman, Fanslow, McMahon, & Shelley, 1999). The category "Threat of Physical or Sexual Violence" is defined as follows: "The use of words, gestures, or weapons to communicate the intent to cause death, disability, injury, or physical harm. Also the use of words, gestures, or weapons to communicate the intent to compel a person to engage in sex acts of abusive sexual contact when the person is either unwilling or unable to consent." Threatening to harm, or harming, a family pet should certainly be cited within this description, yet it is not. No mention is made of the way in which family pets are frequently are used to threaten or coerce victims, despite documentation of this practice (Boat, 1995; Davidson, 1998.)

In addition to the category of "Threat of Physical or Sexual Violence," animal abuse could, and should, be included in the examples used to illustrate the category "Psychological/emotional abuse." Multiple examples are given to illustrate that category, e.g., humiliating the victim, getting the victim to engage in illegal activities, threatening loss of custody of children, smashing objects or destroying property. Again, threats to harm, or the actual harming, of a family pet is not cited as an example of a way in which psychological/emotional abuse could occur.

Federal agencies establish the conceptual framework by which a problem is examined, data is collected, and responses are designed. The framework that is created also influences academic researchers, policy makers, and program planners. The omission of animal cruelty as a form of family violence in the CDC guidebook for researchers could result in missed opportunities to make earlier interventions and offer greater protection to families, including the animals in them.

Child abuse and neglect. Child abuse and neglect is another area in which the federal government keeps databases so that policymakers, researchers, and others can track trends, better understand the nature of the problem, and propose more effective interventions for this fundamental area of public concern. The Children's Bureau in the Administration for Children and Families maintains the national data collection and analysis program, the "National Child Abuse and Neglect Data System Child File (NCANDS)" (Administration for Children and Families, 2006).

One section of the questionnaire in the NCANDS file addresses caretaker risk factors, asking about substance abuse, mental health or physical disability, emotional disturbance, domestic violence, financial strain, and inadequate housing. The identification of caretaker risk factors supports the earlier identification of children and families at risk. Once again, questions about animal cruelty, although potentially quite useful, are not included. For example, information gained from the earlier study cited (Walton-Moss et al., 2005) that found that one of four risk factors for individuals becoming batterers was animal abuse can assist in the earlier identification of family violence. Similarly, including a question on caregiver risk factors about animal cruelty could provide useful information that would allow agencies to make earlier identifications and also make determinations on level of risk a caregiver represents.

State Legislation

In many ways, states are ahead of the federal government, as can be witnessed by the rapid expansion of felony provisions in state animal cruelty laws–from seven states in 1990 to 42 states and the District of Columbia in 2006. With enhanced knowledge, there have been more sophisticated, and inclusive, approaches to family violence and crime in general. It is one that recognizes the patterns and interactions between different types of violent and criminal behavior, e.g., between child abuse and domestic violence, animal abuse and both child and domestic violence, the link between illegal drugs and animal fighting and gangs.

In the past 10 years, there is more attention being paid to the significance of, and effect on, children witnessing violence, in particular, family violence. Prior to this awareness, little notice was given to the very real effects that witnessing, or being in the presence of, such violence had on other family members. That has changed. Resources and attention have been devoted to understanding the effect on children who witness violence at home, and the findings are significant. Children who witness family violence are at a much greater risk of exhibiting aggression or anxiety (Friday, 1995; McCloskey, Figueredo, & Koss, 2005; Osofsky, 1995).[1]

At the state level, Massachusetts House Bill 898, "Subjecting Children to Animal Cruelty," would impose severe sanctions against any person who commits or simulates the killing, torture, or mutilation of an animal in the presence of a child age 18 or under (The Humane Society of the United States, 2006). Two similar bills were introduced in Maryland. One would have increased the penalties for any individual found guilty of committing acts of violence in the presence of a minor; in this legislation animal cruelty was not specifically cited as an example of violence. The other bill had a similar intent, but was focused on animal cruelty as the violent act. It would have increased the penalties for animal cruelty if a minor witnessed animal abuse. Neither bill passed this session of the Maryland General Assembly, however, their introduction demonstrates that there is a more sophisticated understanding of the effects of violence, whether one is the subject of it, or the witness to it.

Other state legislatures have responded by considering legislation that would mandate cross-reporting of animal cruelty and child abuse. This legislation recognizes the benefit of formalizing interactions between animal cruelty investigators and child protective services personnel. Legislation in New York was introduced that would establish cross-reporting of animal cruelty and child abuse, noting "it is essential that those who respond to animal abuse and those who respond to family violence are aware of the connection between violence toward animals and violence toward humans. Cross-reporting helps everyone concerned to work together to establish a coordinated response" (The Humane Society of the United States, 2006). The States of Michigan and Tennessee also are considering similar legislation. Recently, West Virginia signed into law a bill that requires law enforcement officers who are investigating domestic violence to report animal abuse to humane officers, if suspected (The Humane Society of the United States, 2006).

Even without formal legislation, inter-agency agreements can encourage humane officers and child protective service workers to share relevant information. Additionally, both animal services personnel and child protection professionals can be provided with cross-training, so that they are sensitized about the issue and feel competent to make a referral. In addition to legislation, and formal agreements between human service and animal service agencies, the sharing of information can be accomplished on an informal basis. One example of such sharing can be found in Frederick County, Maryland. The animal control officers there have been trained to look for signs of child abuse and domestic violence when they are visiting families on animal-related matters, and, if suspicious, the appropriate humane service agencies. Heartly House, the Frederick area domestic violence shelter, keeps in contact with animal services and will contact endangered women who have been referred to them by the animal service personnel. An added benefit of this sharing of information between animal service and the human services community is that professionals who work in the human service area become more aware of the important link between animal cruelty and family violence.

Professional standards. Standards for education, training, and recertification of mental health professionals and the delivery of mental health services are maintained by the professional groups themselves and also by state agencies. Professional associations, such as the American Psychological Association, the National Association of Social Workers, American Association of Marriage & Family Therapists, and the American Counseling Association help shape the requirements needed to become a licensed mental health professional as well as for maintaining licensure. In addition to the core requirements, State Boards and professional associations may add training or recertification requirements on particular topics, such as substance abuse, ethics, and domestic violence.

Professional standards are developed for good reason: to ensure that mental health professionals are adequately trained in the topics for which they provide treatment. At one time, domestic violence, as an area of study, was not established; health care professionals were not trained to ask questions about the possibility of domestic violence, and there were no programs developed to treat domestic violence victims and batterers. Once recognized as a serious societal problem, however, we witnessed the development of a variety of training and treatment programs related to domestic violence and professional standards established for them. Currently, no states have continuing education requirements for mental health professionals that mention training in the assessment and treatment of animal cruelty.

California licensed psychologists must renew their licenses every two years and during that time are required to complete 36 hours of continuing education for renewal. Three specific courses are required for continuing education: four hours on the laws and ethics for each renewal period; a one-time requirement for a course on spousal or partner abuse assessment, detection, and intervention strategies; and another one-time requirement to complete a three hour course in aging and long-term care (California Board of Psychology, 2006). Psychologists in Florida are required to complete a total of 40 hours of CE every two years. Included in the mandatory 40 hours of CE credits is one hour of domestic violence, two hours of medical errors prevention, and three hours of professional ethics.

Other states, however, such as Colorado, Connecticut, Illinois, and Michigan have no continuing education requirements for psychologists; the continuing requirements in Delaware vary by professional group. Social workers are mandated to take continuing education courses that address substance abuse, while psychologists and professional counselors of mental health have no specific course requirements.

One influence on changes to professional education and training so that they address training in the assessment and treatment of animal cruelty may originate at the federal level. As noted by the National Task Force to End Sexual and Domestic Violence Against Women, the passage of the Violence Against Women Act (VAWA) in 1994, and its reauthorization since, ". . . has changed the landscape for victims who once suffered in silence . . . and a new generation of families and justice system professionals have come to understand that domestic violence, dating violence, sexual assault and stalking are crimes that our society will not tolerate" (The National Task Force to End Sexual and Domestic Violence Against Women, 2005, p. 1).

As noted earlier, empirical evidence supports this claim: the rate of family violence fell between 1993 and 2002 from an estimated 5.4 victims to 2.1 victims per 1,000 U. S. residents age 12 or older (Durose et al., 2005). Although any domestic violence is too much, there has been a notable decrease in the rate of its occurrence. New systems responses were created by VAWA, which created a federal leadership role, encouraged community-coordinated responses between key agencies, recognized and supported the efforts of domestic violence responders, and defined the crimes of domestic violence, dating violence, sexual assault and stalking, as well as identified the promising practices to respond to these crimes. Explicitly stating in a federal statute that "animal cruelty is a crime that our society will not tolerate" would encourage the development of similar responses and ensure that all types of violence in a family receive attention.

Emanating from this focused approach to combat domestic violence was the emergence of batterer intervention programs. These programs have grown into a distinct field of treatment, with training required for practitioners and specific requirements needed for programs to be certified. Every state provides some type of oversight to ensure standards for programs and training for practitioners. In Michigan, standards for batterer intervention were created by the Governor's Task Force on Batterer Intervention Standards (Michigan Domestic Violence Prevention and Treatment Board, 1998). These standards contain great specificity about requirements for program content and structure, including curriculum, modality (use of groups, group size, group facilitation, and mixed gender groups, contra-indicated modalities) and methods (e.g., anger management, couple counseling); completion criteria for contractual discharge; and criteria for noncompliance discharge.

The responsible agency for oversight of batterer intervention programs varies by state. The Massachusetts Department of Health developed guidelines and standards for the certification of batterer intervention programs, which includes standards for intake and evaluation, intervention methodology, educational standards for program staffing, discharge criteria, and more (The Commonwealth of Massachusetts, 1995). In some jurisdictions, such as Los Angeles, the County Probation Department maintains the standards for batterer intervention programs (Los Angeles County Probation Department, 1999).

Unfortunately, unlike batterer intervention, there are no local or state agencies that are responsible for overseeing the development and delivery of mental health services related to the treatment of animal cruelty. This lack of standard setting potentially can exacerbate the problem of animal cruelty. Reviews of youth violence programs found that occasionally, some programs made the problem they were trying to redress worse (Kazdin, 1995). Because of the similarity and overlap in etiology and treatment between children with conduct disorder and children who engage in animal cruelty, it is clear that empirically-based standards need to be constructed for animal cruelty treatment programs. Otherwise, the services provided could have either no effect, or the opposite effect from the one intended.

As yet, the American Psychological Association and the National Association of Social Workers have not recognized that the assessment and treatment of animal cruelty is an emerging treatment area and that this new area demands the same type of guidance and standards as previous emerging treatment areas, such as batterer intervention programs, substance abuse, post-traumatic stress, and others. The American Psychological Association supported the development of a curriculum on partner abuse and relationship violence, which was designed for undergraduates and graduates. The "Intimate Partner Abuse and Relationship Violence Working Group," which was comprised of members from five divisions of the American Psychological Association, observed, "If no specific questions are asked regarding relationship violence, then it is highly likely that important issues will not be treated" (American Psychological Association, no date, p. 36). Until the professional organizations of psychologists, psychiatrists, social workers, and other mental health professionals delineate the importance of asking specific questions about the role and treatment of pets in the family, many professionals will not inquire. As noted, if the question is not asked, the treatment will not be offered, and the problem will continue.

Currently there is a clear trend in state legislation to include provisions in animal cruelty legislation that either mandates, or suggests, treatment for animal cruelty, especially when juveniles are involved. There are now 27 states that contain a counseling provision for juveniles. Regrettably, there also is another trend: these laws are being crafted so that they specify the treatment *before* an assessment is made, and many specifically mention "anger management" as the type of treatment that should be ordered by the court. Interestingly, "anger management" is specifically *excluded* in the specifications for batterer intervention programs.

There can be a number of reasons why an individual is cruel to an animal; a problem with anger is only one, and assumptions should never be made about the cause. Similarly, some programs that developed to respond to bullying in schools assumed that self esteem must be the major factor causing a child to bully. In fact, children who are bullies often have inflated self esteem and need help in making more realistic assessments of themselves.

Until the relevant professional associations recognize the significance of animal abuse, in particular its significance in understanding and treating family violence, the responsibility for shaping professional standards and identifying assessment and intervention options are being developed by individuals outside the field of mental health.

DIRECTIONS FOR CHANGE

Researchers, policy makers, and practitioners are opening the conceptual lens with which family violence is viewed, whether it is child maltreatment or intimate partner violence, so that *all* forms of family violence are captured in that picture. This can be seen in the current trend to report statistics on "family violence" rather than domestic violence and child abuse separately. It also can be seen in the world of legal scholarship in which propositions have been advanced to admit evidence of animal abuse in criminal trials for child and domestic violence (Campbell, 2002) and including animals in protective orders (Gentry, 2001). As seen in the earlier discussion, states are now beginning to adopt legislation that adds pets in the household to protection orders. Other expansions of the role of animals in family life could also be folded into legal definitions of family violence, for example, including pets in the definition of "interfamilial violence" that is used to secure protection orders.

This emerging holistic approach to family violence is encouraging. Thus far, however, there has been no systematic approach to the integration of the treatment of animals into family violence paradigms at the state, federal, or professional levels. Government and professional responses to family violence will be hampered and incomplete until this oversight is corrected and questions about animals in family and community life are incorporated into policy, research, and practice in the field.

A systematic survey is recommended of all federal agencies responsible for the collection of crime data, as well as the collection of data on child abuse and neglect, intimate partner violence, as well as data on youth behavior and lifestyle, to ensure that questions about the treatment of animals are incorporated into the questionnaires in a way that allows retrievable data (Randour, 2004). Professional associations for the mental health profession at the national and state level could benefit by updating their education and training requirements, as well as the requirements for re-licensure, to ensure that they include recent data on the significant role animals play in child development and family life. In order to fulfill the important function of professional standard setting and quality control, state agencies and professional societies need to recognize the emerging field of the assessment and treatment of animal cruelty, both for juveniles and adults.

Shifts in policies and professional standards, however, will take time. In the meantime, any professional who comes into contact with children and families can take steps to include animal-related questions into screening instruments. There also is an urgent reason not to wait before official sanction is given to ask questions about animals. Youth violence has declined, but there are disturbing trends. The juvenile justice system has seen a steep increase in the number of child delinquents, i.e., offenders younger than age 13. Youth referred to juvenile court before the age of 13 are far more likely to become chronic juvenile offenders than youth whose initial contact comes at an earlier age (Loeber, Farrington, & Petechuk, 2003).

We also know from research that animal cruelty may be one of the first signs to indicate that a child is developing deviant and delinquent behavior, and that the median age for diagnosed animal cruelty is 6.5 years of age (Frick et al., 1993). In addition to providing expanded protection to animals, which is in and of itself a worthy goal, the systematic inclusion of animal-related questions into all systems that serve children and families would offer an important tool for detecting pathological development earlier. This would result in enhanced opportunities to offer effective and earlier interventions.

There are several extant instruments that focus exclusively on animal-related experiences that could be used for reference by those interested in incorporating animal-related questions. The Boat Inventory of Animal-Related Experiences is a semi-structured inventory, which is useful in clinical settings. It provides in-depth information about a child's relationship with an animal (Boat, 1995). Another instrument, designed to measure animal maltreatment, is a semi-structured interview for children and their parents, the Children and Animal Assessment Instrument (CAAI), developed by Frank Ascione (1997). The CAAI is very thorough, assessing several dimensions of cruelty to animals, such as severity, frequency, duration, and level of empathy. Because it requires extensive time to administer and to code answers, its use may be limited to research and clinical settings.

A promising new instrument is the P.E.T. Scale for the Measurement of Physical and Emotional Tormenting against Animals. It has the advantage of being a self-administered 9-item scale that measures indirect as well as direct animal abuse. The shortness of the test and the ease of administration make it potentially more useful to a wider audience (Baldry, 2003).

Animals play a vital role in child development, as well as in family and community life. The sooner we recognize that this is the case, and integrate that awareness into our policies and professional standards, the better it will be for all members of the community, including animals.

NOTE

1. A quick review of the many federal initiatives targeted at identifying and helping children who have been exposed to violence demonstrates the importance of this phenomenon. The National Youth Violence Prevention Resource Center (www.safeyouth.

org), which acts as a repository for such information, lists the following organizations or resources under the topic "Witnessing Violence": National Center for Children Exposed To Violence (www.nccev.org); Silent Realities: Supporting Young Children and Their Families Who Experience Violence (www.cwresource.org/hotTopics/ silentRealities/SR.htm); Breaking the Cycle of Violence: Recommendations to Improve the Criminal Justice Response to Child Victims and Witnesses (www.ojd. usdoj.gov/ovc/publications/factshts/pdftxt/monograph.pdf); Children Exposed to Violence: Criminal Justice Resources (www.ojp.usdoj.gov/ovc/publications/factshts/ pdftxt/cevcjr.pdf); Assessing the Exposure of Urban Youth to Violence (www.ncjrs. org/pdffiles/exposure.pdf); Safe from the Start: The National Summit on Children Exposed to Violence (www.ncjrs.org/pdffiles1/ojjdp/182789.pdf); Violence and Young Children's Development (www.eric.ed.gov/contentdelivery/servlet/ERICServlet? accno=ED369578); and Early Childhood Violence Prevention (www.eric.ed.gov/ contentdelivery/servlet/ERICServlet?accno=ED424032).

AUTHOR NOTE

Dr. Mary Lou Randour is a psychologist who was a practicing clinician for 17 years. She received post-graduate training at the Cambridge Hospital at Harvard Medical School and the Washington Psychoanalytic Institute and holds the position of Adjunct Assistant Professor of Psychiatry at the Uniformed Services University of the Health Services. Dr. Randour offers training seminars to law enforcement and court personnel, mental health professionals, educators, animal control and humane society officers, and advocates for domestic violence victims and child protective service workers. The training seminars address the link between animal abuse and human violence as well as the assessment and treatment of animal abuse committed by children and adults.

In addition to offering workshops and seminars, Dr. Randour identifies legislative and policy opportunities that address this important link and organizes efforts in support of them. She is the author of three handbooks: "A Common Bond: Maltreated Children and Animals in the Home" (forthcoming); *AniCare Child: An Assessment and Treatment Approach for Childhood Animal Abuse*; and second author of *The AniCare Model of Treatment for Animal Abuse*, which is designed for use with adults. Dr. Randour also is editor of one book and author of two; her latest book is titled *Animal Grace*.

REFERENCES

Administration for Children and Families. (2006). *National Child Abuse and Neglect Data System Child File*. Retrieved April 15, 2006, from http://www.acf.dhhs.gov/programs/cb/dis/ncands98/record/recorda1.pdf

American Psychological Association. (no date). *Intimate partner abuse and relationship violence*. Washington, DC: Author.

Arluke, A., & Luke, C. (1997). Physical cruelty toward animals in Massachusetts, 1975-1996. *Society and Animals, 5*, 195-204.

Ascione, F. R. (2000). *Safe havens for pets: Guidelines for programs sheltering pets for women who are battered*. Logan, UT: Author.

Ascione, F. R., Thompson, T. M., & Black, T. (1997). Childhood cruelty to animals: Assessing cruelty dimensions and motivations. *Anthrozoos, 10*, 170-179.

Ascione, F. R., Weber, C. V., Thompson, T. M., Heath, J., Maruyama, M., & Hayashi, K. (2007). Battered pets and domestic violence: Animal abuse reported by women experiencing intimate violence and by non-abused women. *Violence Against Women, 13*, 354-373.

Baldry, A. C. (2003). The development of the P.E.T. scale for the measurement of physical and emotional tormenting against animals in adolescents. *Society and Animals, 12*, 235-249.

Boat, B. W. (1995). The relationship between violence to children and violence to animals. *Journal of Interpersonal Violence, 3*, 229-235.

California Board of Psychology. (2006). *Mandatory continuing education requirements.* Retrieved June 1, 2006, from http:www.psychboard.ca.gov/licensing/education.html

Campbell, A. (2002). The admissibility of evidence of animal abuse in criminal trials for child and domestic abuse. *Boston College Law Review, 43*, 2-24.

Center for the Study and Prevention of Violence. (2006). *Blueprints for violence prevention overview.* Retrieved June 1, 2006, from http://www.colorado.edu/cspv/blueprints/

The Commonwealth of Massachusetts, Department of Public Health (1995). *Massachusetts guidelines and standards for the certification of batterer intervention programs.* Boston, MA: Author.

Davidson, H. (1998). The link between animal cruelty and child maltreatment. *Child Law Practice, 3*, 62-64.

DeViney, E., Dickert, J., & Lockwood, R. (1983). The care of pets within child abusing families. *International Journal for the Study of Animal Problems, 4*, 321-329.

Durose, M. R., Harlow, C. W., Langan, P. A., Motivans, M., Rantala, R. R., & Smith, E. L. (2005, June). *Family violence statistics: Including statistics on strangers and acquaintances.* Washington, DC: U. S. Department of Justice, NCJ 207846.

Edelson, J. L. (1999, February). The overlap between child maltreatment and women battering. *Violence Against Women, 5*, 124-54.

Flores, J. R. (2003). Juveniles in court. *Juvenile Offenders and Victims National Report Series Bulletin.* Washington, DC: U. S. Department of Justice, Office of Juvenile Justice and Delinquency Prevention, NCJ 195420.

Florida Psychological Association. (2006). *Continuing education requirements.* Retrieved June 1, 2006, from http://www.flapsych.com/displaycommon.cfm?an=1&subarticlenbr=88

Frick, P. J., VanHorn, Y., Lahey, B. B., Christ, M. A. G., Loeber, R., Hart, E. A., et al. (1993). Oppositional defiant disorder and conduct disorder: A meta-analytic review of factor analyses and cross-validation in a clinical sample. *Clinical Psychology Review, 13*, 319-350.

Friday, J. C. (1995). The psychological impact of violence in underserved communities. *Journal of Health Care for the Poor and Underserved, 6*, 503-409.

Gentry, D. J. (2001). Including companion animals in protective orders: Curtailing the reach of domestic violence. *Yale Journal of Law and Feminism, 13*, 1-20.

The Humane Society of the United States. (2006). *Subjecting children to animal cruelty; Massachusetts House Bill 898.* Retrieved June 1, 2006, from http:www.hsus.org/legislation_laws/state_legislation/massachusetts/ma

The Humane Society of the United States. (2006). *State legislation: New York.* Retrieved June 1, 2006, from http:www.hsus.org/legislation_laws/state_legislation/new_york

The Humane Society of the United States. (2006). *State legislation: West Virginia.* Retrieved June 1, 2006, from http:www.hsus.org/legislation_laws/state_legislation/west_virginia/wv

Kazdin, A. E. (1995). Interventions for aggressive and antisocial children. In L. Eron, J. Gentry, & P. Schlegel (Eds.), *Reason for hope: A psychosocial perspective on violence and youth* (pp. 341-382). Washington, DC: American Psychological Association.

Kelley, B. T., Loeber, R., Keenan, K., & DeLamaatre, M. (1997, December). Developmental pathways in boys' disruptive and delinquent behavior. *Office of Juvenile Justice and Delinquency Prevention Bulletin:* U. S. Department of Justice.

Loeber, R. (2004). *The Pittsburgh study.* Annual Conference on Criminal Justice Research and Evaluation. Department of Justice, Washington, DC.

Loeber, R., Farrington, D. P., & Petechuk, D. (2003). Child delinquency: Early intervention and prevention. *Office of Juvenile Justice and Delinquency Prevention: Child Delinquency Bulletin.* Washington, DC: U. S. Department of Justice.

Los Angles County Probation Department. (1999, July). Approved batterers' programs. 76B77-P10010(REV 7/99)

McCloskey, L. A., Figueredo, A. J., & Koss, M. (1995). The effects of systematic family violence on children's health. *Child Development, 66,* 1239-1261.

McKinney, C., Sieger, K., Agliata, A. K., & Renk, K. (2005). Children's exposure to domestic violence: Striving toward an ecological framework for intervention. *Journal of Emotional Abuse, 6,* 1-23.

Michigan Domestic Violence Prevention and Treatment Board. (1998). *Batterer intervention standards for the State of Michigan.* Lansing, MI: Author.

The National Task Force to End Sexual and Domestic Violence Against Women. (2005). *The Violence Against Women Act:10 years of progress and moving forward.* Washington, DC: Author.

Office of Juvenile Justice and Delinquency Prevention. (2006). *Compendium of National Juvenile Justice Data Sets.* Retrieved June 1, 2006, from http://ojjdp.ncjrs.org/ojstatbb/Compendium/asp/Compendium.asp?selData=3

Osofsky, J. D. (1995). The effects of exposure to violence on young children. *American Psychologist, 9,* 782-788.

Randour, M. L. (2004). Including animal cruelty as a factor in assessing risk and designing interventions. Washington, DC: *Proceedings of Persistently Safe Schools,* 103-110.

Renner, L. M., & Slack, K. S. (2004). Intimate partner violence and child maltreatment: Understanding co-occurrence and intergenerational connections. Discussion Paper no. 1278-04, Institute for Research on Poverty. Available at: http://www.ssc.wisc.edu/irp/

Saltzman, L. E., Fanslow, J. L., McMahon, P. M., & Shelley, G. A. (1999). *Intimate partner violence surveillance: Uniform definitions and recommended data elements, Version 1.0.* Atlanta, GA: National Center for Injury Prevention and Control, Centers for Disease Control and Prevention.

Snyder, H. (2005, August). Juvenile arrests 2003. *Juvenile Justice Bulletin*. Washington, DC: U.S. Department of Justice, Office of Juvenile Justice and Delinquency Prevention.

Walton-Moss, B. J., Mangannelo, J., Frye, V., & Campbell, J. (2005). Risk factors for intimate partner violence and associated injury among urban women. *Journal of Community Health, 30*, 377-389.

doi:10.1300/J135v07n03_06

Cisco's Kids:
A Pet Assisted Therapy
Behavioral Intervention Program

Gary P. Cournoyer
Clarissa M. Uttley

SUMMARY. Cisco's Kids is an intervention program designed to address behavioral and social difficulties of incarcerated youth at the Rhode Island Training School. Incorporating principles of Professional Pet Assisted Therapy (PPAT), the first author developed the program based around working with his chocolate Labrador retriever, Cisco. This article details the design, goals, and results of the program over a period of two and one-half years. During this time, over 50 students ages 13-18 participated in the Cisco's Kids program. This program has collected qualitative data over the course of its existence, which provides support that this program has a positive effect on the participants. Authors also discuss a brief history of Pet Assisted Therapy (PAT) and the future of the Cisco's Kids program as well as a newly developed college-level course in PAT. doi:10.1300/J135v07n03_07 *[Article copies available for a fee from The Haworth Document Delivery Service: 1-800-HAWORTH. E-mail address: <docdelivery@haworthpress.com> Website: <http://www.HaworthPress. com> © 2007 by The Haworth Press. All rights reserved.]*

Address correspondence to: Gary P. Cournoyer (E-mail: gcournoyer@nccmhc. org).

[Haworth co-indexing entry note]: "Cisco's Kids: A Pet Assisted Therapy Behavioral Intervention Program." Cournoyer, Gary P., and Clarissa M. Uttley. Co-published simultaneously in *Journal of Emotional Abuse* (The Haworth Maltreatment & Trauma Press, an imprint of The Haworth Press) Vol. 7, No. 3, 2007, pp. 117-126; and: *Animal Abuse and Family Violence: Linkages, Research, and Implications for Professional Practice* (ed: Marti T. Loring, Robert Geffner, and Janessa Marsh) The Haworth Maltreatment & Trauma Press, an imprint of The Haworth Press, 2007, pp. 117-126. Single or multiple copies of this article are available for a fee from The Haworth Document Delivery Service [1-800-HAWORTH, 9:00 a.m. - 5:00 p.m. (EST). E-mail address: docdelivery@haworthpress.com].

KEYWORDS. Pet assisted therapy, incarcerated youth, students

INTRODUCTION

As far back as the early Greeks and Romans, the importance of the bond between humans and animals was known to be special. Numerous articles have been written about research conducted on the positive nature of the human-animal bond (e.g., Jalongo, Astorino, & Bomboy, 2004; Rud & Beck, 2000; Stengle, 2005). Psychologist Boris M. Levinson (1969) was one of the first clinicians to notice the difference in his clients when he brought his dog Jingles to his office. In one situation, a child who previously had been non-verbal during his office visits became more open when Jingles was present. This experience caused Levinson to explore the possible benefits of having a pet present during sessions with his clients.

A study conducted by Barbara J. Wood (2001) looked at elementary school children diagnosed as Severe Behavior Disordered. These children were found to behaviorally improve by 8% and their attendance rate increased by over 10% when their therapy was pet assisted. Other research has shown that troubled teenagers are more likely to open up in sessions when a therapist brings a dog (Bardill & Hutchinson, 1997; Parshall, 2003). At times, the youth would express their feelings through the dog, i.e., "your dog looks sad."

A study by Gonski, Peacock, and Ruckert (1986) as cited in Linda Nebbe's 1991 book, *Nature as a Guide*, compared the responses during the intake process of juvenile offenders entering a residential facility when the interviewer had her dog present and when she did not. The results showed that in every case where the dog was present, the young men responded with more openness and less hostility than in interviews when the dog was not present. Debra Phillips Parshall (2003), a grief counselor who utilized a little dog named Rudy in some of her counseling sessions, stated that Rudy provided a means of connecting with these children. She also stated that Animal Assisted Therapy (AAT) has been beneficial in attaining the goals of counseling in these situations.

Finally, Bardill and Hutchinson (1997) discuss the operant conditioning that took place between Graham, their therapy pet, and the patients involved. Graham would respond positively to acts of kindness many times during the day. Negative behaviors towards Graham were responded to by avoidance. Thus, negative behaviors would be extinguished through negative reinforcement.

THE CISCO'S KIDS PROGRAM

Building on the literature suggesting that working with animals builds a bridge between the counselor and troubled youth, the Cisco's Kids Program was developed. Cisco's Kids is a Professional Pet Assisted Therapy (PPAT) Program developed by Gary Cournoyer, MSW, LICSW, the school social worker in the Rhode Island Training School's education program, which is known as the Youth Career Education Center (YCEC). This PPAT program is conducted in this facility with the assistance of Cisco, who is Cournoyer's 9-year-old chocolate Labrador retriever and the therapy pet in this program.

The program assists incarcerated youth ages 13-18 who manifest serious behavioral problems within the education program. These behaviors have a negative impact on both the students' and their classmates' ability to learn. Cisco's Kids is a voluntary program offered to all incarcerated youth at the YCEC. Of all the students recommended for Cisco's Kids, only one student chose not to take part due to the fact that he had heard from his attorney that he may be getting out shortly. The involvement of family court that released some students early and the fact that some of the students left before their end of sentence for a community placement were the only reasons students who started the group did not complete the cycle. The parents/guardians of these youth gave their consent for their children to be in this voluntary program, which consists of two types of therapeutic intervention.

The first and main therapeutic intervention is through group professional pet assisted therapy, while the second intervention is through individual pet assisted therapy. The individual sessions are provided for students who are not behaviorally able to function in a group environment. Both interventions are designed to improve the student's behavioral performance within this academic setting. Due to the two different methods of intervention, the results presented below do not include the participants receiving individual sessions.

GOALS OF CISCO'S KIDS

Goals for the Cisco's Kids program were developed in consultation with the clinical social workers, the principal of the education program, other administrators, and incarcerated youth of the Rhode Island Training School. Input from all of the above parties assisted in the development and implementation of the following goals:

1. To help the students to improve their behavior within this academic program by developing self-respect.
2. To help the students to improve their social skills by interacting amongst themselves (group), the Clinician, and the pet in an acceptable manner.
3. To provide an atmosphere of unconditional love resulting in an improvement in the students' self-esteem.
4. To explain to the students that all living things have feelings to assist them in developing a respect for pets, themselves, and each other, as well as everyone they interact with.
5. To provide a stress-free environment where the students will be more comfortable to discuss issues in their own lives and how these may be impacting on their behavior within the school program.
6. To help the students learn how to react to conflict and stressful situations in a more pro-social manner.

Program Methodology

The Cisco's Kids Program currently takes place in the Youth Career Education Center on Fridays. In the mornings, there are two groups and, at times, one individual session scheduled. The groups have a maximum of six students, thus the Cisco's Kids program has approximately 13 students participating each week. Students have the option of continuing in future groups or ending their participation after attending only one set of sessions. All of these students have volunteered and been referred by their teachers or clinical social workers, and all have histories of significant behavior problems in school settings. The students are also asked to fill out questionnaires concerning their experiences with animals. Some of the students involved in the groups have admitted to some abuse of animals in the past. This does not exclude them from taking part in Cisco's Kids; however, these students are interviewed to insure that Cisco would not be at risk should they join the groups. The groups are designed to be open-ended, which means that as one student leaves another may join. The length of each session is one class period of one hour.

At the beginning of each session, the school social worker reviews with the members how they have behaved in the past week in school. This is accomplished by reviewing the students' school points, any written sanctions for more serious behaviors, and teacher feedback. Students can receive a maximum of 20 points per week in school. Students who have had some behavioral difficulties during the past week are asked to review the circumstances of these occurrences. They are then asked to brainstorm other ways they could have reacted in these situations. If they have difficulties doing this, other members of the group are asked to assist. Students must take responsibility for their difficulties. They are not allowed to blame teachers or classmates. Students are also encouraged to discuss other issues that may be impacting negatively on their education. This may involve other issues at the training school, family issues, concerns about their upcoming release, and problems with relationships or anything else that may be bothering them. There also is a curriculum in place that has the students look at their goals while at the training school and at different times of their lives.

While this is taking place, Cisco can be seen walking around the room, interacting with different students who may pet him or bend down so he can kiss them. At times, the students pick up Cisco's ball and throw it for him. He will roll it or throw it back. During the last five minutes of these sessions, the students are allowed to give Cisco treats and learn how to have Cisco do some of his tricks. As the sessions progress, Cisco's connection with the members of the groups also progresses. Some of the students who in the beginning were not willing to interact with him become much more comfortable with him in the later sessions (e.g., they are much more likely to get on the floor and play with him).

In the afternoons, Cisco is in the school social worker's office and meets students on an individual basis who are there for assistance with any number of issues. Cisco is also in the halls with the school social worker when students arrive in the morning and after lunch and when students leave before lunch and at the end of the day. This allows many students to interact with Cisco. All students who stop to pet him leave with a smile on their face. Also, students who just watch other students interact start to smile. Cisco also visits many other areas of the training school such as the medical clinic, the records room, and the Educational Transition Office. Employees look forward to these visits. The Superintendent has even said that Cisco appears to bring a sense of normalcy to the prison setting.

Program Results

As of this writing, the Cisco's Kids Program has completed six cycles and has seen over 50 students graduate from the program. Behavioral changes have been assessed using a pre- and post-group comparison of points earned in the education program. For the students who were in the first cycle, which was nine weeks, it was found that the group members' school points had improved an average of 26%. For the second cycle, the group members' school points improved by an average of 13%. This same information was reviewed for the members of the third and the fourth cycles; the school points of the group members improved by an average of over 10% for the third cycle and by over 14% for the fourth cycle.

The fifth cycle was comprised of one group of boys and one group of girls. The girls' group was geared more toward social skills development than behavioral development because of the numerous problems they had getting along in their current living situations. For this cycle of the boys' group, there was not sufficient data because a number of them left early and were replaced by new members, leaving only two original group members to complete this six-week cycle.

Of importance to note: the results of this cycle identified a difference in the dynamics between the boys' and the girls' PPAT groups. Consistently, the boys in the group have been very physical with Cisco. They wanted to play with him and his toy, usually resulting in their chasing him around the classroom. In the girls' group, the females were much more loving and caring than the boys. They wanted to calmly pet and hug Cisco and have him give them kisses, and there was very little playing, chasing, and physical horseplay.

The sixth cycle had many repeat group members. At the end of this cycle, the students' points did not show any significant improvement, but it should be noted that there was also no decrease in the average of their school points. One reason for this lack of improvement could be that most of the group members had completed at least one previous cycle and had already shown significant improvement in their school points.

DISCUSSION

The fact that the majority of students who completed at least one cycle of Cisco's Kids did show a noteworthy improvement in their functioning within the education program is a very positive result. This is also evidenced by the fact that there have been numerous positive comments by some of the students' teachers as to how they see improvement in their behavior and attitude. Some of the students have also spoken about their experiences in this program. One student said that he felt that Cisco really listens when he speaks. Another student, when asked about this program, said that "you get to talk about your problems in this group and you get to help other students with theirs. Cisco makes it easier to do this." Several of the students commented that it was easier to discuss problems with the social worker when Cisco was in the room. Conversations would take place over ball tossing with Cisco or while students where petting Cisco. There also develops a caring for Cisco among a number of the group members. An example of this is when a student asked to use the bathroom. When he returned, he had four little cups filled with water. He asked if he could put them in Cisco's bowl since he had noticed his water getting low. Notably, this student initially did not want to engage Cisco at all.

During each one of the group cycles, the topic of manhood versus fatherhood is discussed. It usually happens early in the sessions when one of the boys notices that Cisco has been neutered. They usually question why I would take away his manhood by not allowing him to have puppies. They are appalled that I would make him "less of man." This always leads to a good discussion on how being a man is not necessarily connected to having children. Also, we discuss the issue of the large number of unwanted pets that are euthanized yearly because of people's failure to neuter and spay their pets.

Cisco's main achievement is to create a bridge between the students and the school social worker. He gives all group members unconditional love and helps to break down the walls and barriers that many of these students have built over the years. A collateral effect of this program is that the group members begin to have much more contact outside of the groups with the school social worker. They seem to be much more willing to remove themselves from stressful situations and to try to resolve these situations in a more appropriate manner with the school social worker's assistance. A major example of this was when there were some serious gang problems surfacing in the education program. These problems manifested themselves in a significant number of fights in the education program in a two-week period. Two of the group members met with the school social worker because they were concerned about this and wanted to know what they could do about it. After a lengthy discussion, with Cisco present, the two group members provided a list of 13 names of the students who were involved in this gang situation. The school social worker and a Deputy Superintendent met with all students named. Cisco was also present and engaged all of these students. After a long and at times heated discussion, all students present agreed to end the conflicts. There were no further problems noted from this conflict following this meeting.

It should also be noted that since the beginning of this program in July 2004, approximately 50 students from the education program in the Rhode Island Training School have graduated from the PPAT Program and been released as of this writing. Of those 50 students, only two of them have been re-sentenced since the completion of their participating in the Cisco's Kids program. This paper is a presentation of a professional pet assisted therapy program developed based on the needs of a population, which the first author worked with on a daily basis. It should be made clear that this program was constantly adapting to the needs of the population at the Rhode Island Training School, thus the intervention, while consistent in the day of occurrence, consisted of dialogue that was based on the needs of the students.

Cisco's Kids presents a qualitative study of how professional pet assisted therapy may be provided to assist incarcerated youth with social, emotional, and behavioral difficulties. Future work in the field of professional pet assisted therapy needs to be conducted that will provide a more quantitative study of the benefits of these programs to incarcerated youth. It is the hope of the authors that researchers will take up the charge to create and validate instruments that will measure change in behavior based on exposure to professional pet assisted therapy programming. Additionally, future research should be conducted to follow-up with the students completing the Cisco's Kids program. An interview protocol could be created to assess the value of the program to students who have not committed any crimes since leaving the program, and historical data could be accessed through the YCEC to retrieve numbers of participants that have been re-sentenced and the nature of these crimes.

EPILOGUE

At the end of April 2006, Gary Cournoyer retired from State Service after almost 30 years. This ended the Cisco's Kids program as discussed above. Since that time, Cournoyer has started to work at Newport County Community Mental Health Center as an Administrator overseeing the Children's Intensive Services Program. This program works with children from 3-18 years of age who, due to significant psychiatric issues, are at risk of out-of-home placement and possibly psychiatric hospitalization. Cournoyer is working with Human Resources as well as other members of the agency to develop a new Pet Assisted Therapy program utilizing Cisco's talents to hopefully assist this population. The goal is to have this program functioning by summer 2007. Cisco is looking forward to returning to work. Also, in October 2006, Cournoyer taught a one-credit college course at Salve Regina University in Newport, RI on Professional Pet Assisted Therapy. This is believed to be the first PPAT college course for credit taught in Rhode Island. Cisco took part in this class as well as a number of other therapy pets with their facilitators. Feedback from the class has been very positive, encouraging Cournoyer to develop future credit-based PAT courses.

AUTHOR NOTE

Gary P. Cournoyer, MSW, LICSW, is currently employed as an Administrator at Newport County Community Mental Health Center in the Children's Intensive Services Program. He previously worked for over 18 years in Rhode Island's Juvenile prison. Gary is a credentialed Pet Assisted Therapy Facilitator working with his rescued chocolate Labrador retriever, Cisco. With Cisco, Gary and his wife Anne share their home with two other rescue dogs: Shiloh, a 7-year-old Beagle and Daphne, a 2-year-old Beagle-Jack Russell mix. Gary can be reached at: Newport County Community Mental Health Center, 26 Valley Road, Middletown, RI 02842, 401-848-6363, ext.120, gcournoyer@nccmhc.org

Clarissa M. Uttley is a Behavioral Science doctoral student at the University of Rhode Island, where she received an M.S. in Human Development and Family Studies. She is also a credentialed Pet Assisted Therapy Facilitator and works alongside her dog, Nina, at early childhood centers. Clarissa can be reached at: University of Rhode Island, Department of Human Development and Family Studies, 2 Lower College Road, Kingston, RI 02881, 401-874-2150, clarissa@mail.uri.edu

REFERENCES

Bardill, N., & Hutchinson, S. (1997). Animal-assisted therapy with hospitalized adolescents. *Journal of Child and Adolescent Psychiatric Nursing, 10*, 17.

Jalongo, M. R., Astorino, T., & Bomboy, N. (2004). Canine visitors: The influence of therapy dogs on young children's learning and well-being in classrooms and hospitals. *Early Childhood Education Journal, 32*(1), 9-16.

Levinson, B. (1969). *Pet oriented child psychotherapy.* Springfield, IL: Charles C. Thomas Publishers.

Nebbe, L. L. (1991). *Nature as a guide.* Minneapolis, MN: Educational Media Corp.

Parshall, D. P. (2003). Research and reflection: Animal assisted therapy in mental health settings. *Counseling and Values, 48*, 47-56.

Rud, A. G., & Beck, A. M. (2000). Kids and critters in class together. *Phi Delta Kappan, 82*(4), 313-316.

Stengle, J. (2005, November 15). Dogs lower anxiety among heart patients. *The Providence Journal*. Retrieved November 17, 2005, from http://www.projo.com/

Wood, B. J. (2001). The effects of a canine co-therapist on individual therapy sessions with elementary school children with SBH (Severe Behaviorally Handicapped). In P. Salotto, *Assisted therapy: A loving intervention and an emerging profession: Leading to a friendlier, healthier, and more peaceful world* (pp. 11-15). Norton, MA: D. J. Publications.

doi:10.1300/J135v07n03_07

Index

Abuse. *See also* Animal abuse;
 Woman abuse
 case examples of, 34-37
 of children. *See* Child abuse
 children/adolescents experiencing,
  and risk for committing
  animal abuse, 45
 defined, 10
 detecting, 10
 difficulty in defining, 9-10
 experiencing, and committing
  animal abuse, 45
 impact of multiple forms of, 41-42
 multiple forms of, 17
 psychological trauma model of, 33
 survivors of, 33-34
 as victimizing traumas, 42
 of women. *See* Woman abuse
Abused animals. *See also* Pets
 behavioral signs of, 48
 characteristics of, 46-47
 "Safe Haven" programs for, 100
Abused women
 abuse of pets for
  domination/control of, 14
 attachment to pets and, 13-14
 concern over pets and, 21
 pet ownership and, 64-65
 pets as source of emotional support
  for, 65
Abusers
 perception of pets as property and,
  15
 use of pets for domination/control
  and, 14
Acculturation, intimate partner
 violence and, 62
American Humane Association, xviii,3
AniCare Model, 50

Animal abuse. *See also* Pets
 adult motivations for, 3
 assessing children who witness, 44
 assessment instruments for, 112
 case of John Jefferson and, 98
 challenges of defining, 2
 by child/adolescent, as indicative
  for potential for violence
  against people, 45
 children as victims/perpetrators of,
  85-86
 children of domestic violence and
  witnessing, 100-101
 children's motivations for, 3
 crime data collection systems for,
  101-104
 in criminal prosecutions, 99
 defining, with child abuse
  typologies, 47-48
 difficulty in defining, 10-11
 domestic violence and, 65
 empathy and, 3
 empirical evidence of, 11-13
 experiencing abuse and committing, 45
 in families, reasons to address,
  18-21
 family violence and, 84,98-99
 federal policies for, 101-105
 felony-level penalties for, xvii,101
 as form of child maltreatment, 42
 impact of, 42-46
 including questions about, in
  protocol, 21-22
 intimate partner violence and,
  64-66,98,99
 lesbian partner violence and, 13
 link between child abuse and, 11,99
 link between family violence and,
  9,12-13

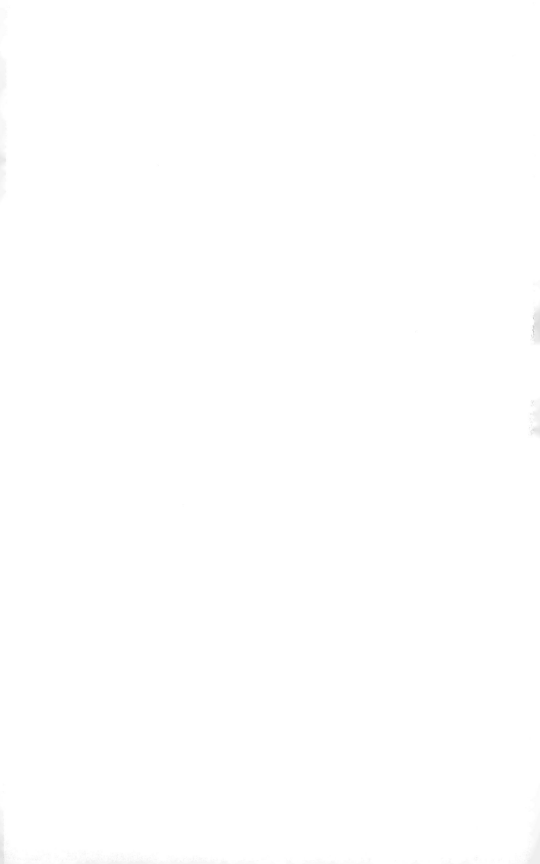

Printed and bound by CPI Group (UK) Ltd, Croydon, CR0 4YY

17/10/2024

01775687-0015